A SHORT HISTORY OF
PSYCHIATRY

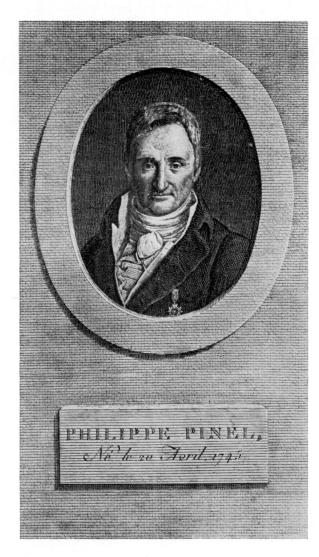

PINEL

A SHORT HISTORY OF PSYCHIATRY

by

ERWIN H. ACKERKNECHT

Professor of the History of Medicine
University of Zürich

Translated from the German by

SULAMMITH WOLFF, M.A. M.R.C.P. D.P.M.

The Maudsley Hospital, London

HAFNER PUBLISHING COMPANY
NEW YORK　:　:　LONDON
1959

CONTENTS

Translator's Note

I would like to express my gratitude to Miss Helen Marshall for reading and correcting the manuscript and for making many valuable suggestions, and to Mrs. Sara Frisby for her secretarial help.

SULAMMITH WOLFF

PREFACE

PSYCHIATRY is more than a medical speciality. 150 years ago it was described by Reil as one of the three basic disciplines of medicine, together with internal medicine and surgery. One might even go further and say that there is no case of illness in which the psychiatrist has not some contribution to make. The social significance of psychiatry, too, can hardly be exaggerated. In the United States, for example, 50% to 70% of available hospital beds are required for mentally ill patients.

Nevertheless, to write the history of psychiatry is an unrewarding task. The psychiatric historian cannot as yet indulge in the paeans of progress and achievement which nowadays usually make the work of his colleague in general medicine so much easier. As Griesinger said a hundred years ago; and his gloomy statement is still unfortunately often true today; we know as little about mental disorders as men knew about diseases of the chest in the days before Laënnec. One is indeed frequently tempted to wonder whether the well-known " historical spiral " is in this case just a simple circular movement. This is, of course, the fault neither of the historians nor of psychiatrists. Psychiatry is the youngest branch of medicine. For historical reasons, which will be more closely examined below, its renaissance occurred two hundred years later than that of the other medical disciplines. In addition, psychiatry still suffers from the hostility which has always been directed against the mentally ill and against their physicians. Above all, psychiatry is concerned with the most difficult medico-physiological problem; that of the body-soul relationship, which has remained unsolved to the present day. Anatomy, physiology, morbid anatomy and chemistry, which have contributed so much to other disciplines during the last hundred years, have been far less helpful in the elucidation of mental illnesses. For this reason large numbers of different and often dogmatic schools continue to exist in psychiatry today, as they existed in internal medicine in earlier times. This increases the difficulties of surveying and of understanding the subject, but is, of course, no reason for abandoning the study of psychiatry or of its history: on the contrary, it makes it perhaps all the more necessary. But it seemed best to point out these difficulties frankly in the hope

i

that the reader will thereby be better enabled to understand both the shortcomings of this book and its subject matter. Indeed, just because progress in psychiatry has been so very slow, study of the past may have more to offer to the psychiatrist of today than to his medical and surgical colleagues.

A further obstacle in the way of writing a short history of psychiatry is the fact that very few basic studies, and even fewer good ones, have been carried out in this field, particularly in recent times. I have, therefore, had to depend primarily upon my own studies of original sources and to present many summaries of texts of the older writers. At the same time, for reasons of space I have had to limit myself in this to the writings of a few men of particular importance. This does not mean that I support the " great men " theory of history. Great men are made possible only by the work of their contemporaries and of their predecessors. If Pinel or Kraepelin or Freud had never lived, others would have carried out their work with greater or lesser distinction. This is not to deny that these great men were the most able representatives of the psychiatry of their day and that they merit the closest study in a short historical review. In reporting the older texts, I have attempted to reproduce the sum total of the opinions expressed in them and have not, as is unfortunately the current trend, merely selected what appears to be modern in them.

I have tried to be as brief as possible and am, therefore, liable to be reproached for various omissions. I am, however, encouraged to hope that because my book is short, it will be read; and this seems to me to be a reasonable aim. Because I wished and needed to be concise, I have had to limit myself to the presentation of only a small selection of the many great names and of the abundant literature of the nineteenth century. In dealing with the twentieth century, however, I have restricted myself still further and have not ventured to do more than touch on its basic trends. This is not only for reasons of space; I am convinced that it is almost impossible for an historian to produce anything of value if he is too close to the period he is studying. As a medical historian I have here concerned myself only with medical psychiatry; although a philosophical psychiatry has been known to exist since the time of the Greeks. The decision to limit myself in this way was relatively easy to make, since it seems to me that philosophical psychiatry has never been of much help in practice. I have perhaps not always shown the proper respect for attempts, so common in the history of psychiatry, to conceal ignorance behind new words and a spurious profundity. It is high time, however, that someone revealed what stuff the emperor's new clothes are made of.

Although, even in the twentieth century, psychiatric achievements have lagged behind those of internal medicine and surgery, the last fifty years have seen the emergence of much that is promising. Psychiatry has always been in many ways the most human and most interesting of the medical sciences. I venture to hope that the reader will find at least a reflection of this in my small book.

I am very grateful to Dr. Joachim Bodamer of Winnental and to Professor Victor Gourevitch of Chicago, for sparing the time to read and criticise my manuscript; despite our basic differences in outlook.

ERWIN H. ACKERKNECHT

Zürich
May, 1957

LIST OF PLATES

BIBLIOGRAPHICAL COMMENTS

WE would like to draw the reader's attention to the following more recent general accounts of the history of psychiatry:

In German

BIRNBAUM, K., *Geschichte der Psychiatrischen Wissenschaft*, in BUMKE, O., *Handbuch der Geisteskrankheiten*, Vol. I, pp. 11-49, Berlin, 1928. de BOOR, W., *Psychiatrische Systematik seit Kahlbaum*, Berlin, 1954. KIRCHHOFF, Th., *Grundriss einer Geschichte der deutschen Irrenpflege*, Berlin, 1890. Idem., *History of Psychiatry*, in ASCHAFFENBURG, G., *Handbuch der Psychiatrie*, Vol. I, pp. 1-48, Vienna, 1912. Idem., *Deutsche Irrenaerzte*, 2 vols., Berlin, 1921 and 1924. KOLLE, K., *Grosse Nervenaerzte*, Stuttgart, 1956. KORNFELD, S., *History of Psychiatry*, in Puschmann's *Handbuch der Geschichte der Medizin*, ed. M. Neuburger and J. Pagel, Vol. IV, pp. 600-728, Jena, 1905. KRAEPELIN, E., *Hundert Jahre der Psychiatrie*. Zscht. ges. Neur. 38, pp. 161-275, 1918. LAEHR, H., *Gedenktage der Psychiatrie*, Berlin, 1899. Idem, *Die Literatur der Psychiatrie, Neurologie und Psychologie von 1459-1799*, 2 vols., Berlin, 1900. SCHULTZ, J. H., *Psychotherapie, Leben und Werke Grosser Aerzte*, Stuttgart, 1952.

We would mention especially the works of Joachim Bodamer and Karl Jaspers, to which reference will be made later.

In English

BROMBERG, W., *Man above Humanity: a History of Psychotherapy*, Philadelphia, 1954. DEUTSCH, A., *The Mentally Ill in America*, New York, 1937. HALL, J. K., etc., Editors, *One Hundred Years of American Psychiatry*, New York, 1944. LEWIS, N., *A Short History of Psychiatry*, New York, 1941. TUKE, D. H., *Chapters on the History of the Insane in the British Isles*, London, 1882. WHITWELL, J. R., *Historical Notes on Psychiatry* (*Early Times to End of 16th Century*), London, 1936. ZILBOORG, G., *History of Medical Psychology*, New York, 1941.

We refer the reader also to articles by Raymond de Saussure (e.g. Journ. Hist. Med. 1, 365-97, 1946; CIBA Symposia, 2nd Series, pp. 1122-1252, 1950) and to those of H. Ellenberger in the *Bulletin of the Menninger Clinic*.

In French

ELLENBERGER, H., *La Psychiatrie Suisse*, Aurillac, 1953. LAIGNEL-
LAVASTINE, M., and VICHON, J., *Les Malades de l'Esprit et leur Médecine
du XVIe au XIXe siècle*, Paris, 1930. SEMELAIGNE, R., *Les Grands
Aliénistes Français*, Paris, 1894. Idem, *Aliénistes et Philanthropes*,
Paris, 1912. Idem, *Les Pionniers de la Psychiatrie Française avant et
après Pinel*, 2 vols., Paris, 1930, 1932. RITTI, A., *Histoire des travaux
de la Société Medico-Psychologique et éloges de ses membres*, 2 vols.,
Paris, 1913, 1914. VIE, J., *Histoire de la Psychiatrie*, in LAIGNEL-
LAVASTINE, *Histoire Générale de la Médecine*, Paris, 1949, Vol. III, pp.
278-322.

CHAPTER I

ETHNOLOGICAL COMMENTS

IN this book we shall be concerned with the history of psychiatry; that is, with the science of mental diseases. We can, therefore, be brief in our discussion of primitive ideas which have no claim to be scientific. The concept of disease held by primitive peoples is totally different from ours. They do not, with a few exceptions,[1] have mental illnesses in our sense. Disease is to them a monistic concept; there is no division between diseases of the body and the mind such as we know, but the nature of disease is the same, whatever the symptoms. Almost all illnesses are attributed to the intervention of supernatural forces; such as evil spirits, gods, witches or magicians. Illnesses of all kinds are frequently explained on the basis of possession by evil spirits, and this is particularly so in the case of mental illnesses. So long as one can believe in spirits this explanation carries conviction. It can help one to understand fairly easily how quantities of strange, obscene and nonsensical material can spring from what, until then, had been a familiar and reasonable human being. One might even ask oneself whether this explanation, which is used by many primitives for all diseases, did not originate from empirical observations made on cases of mental illness.

The methods of treatment used are of the greatest interest to the modern observer. Primitive societies are familiar with several effective drugs and several effective physical methods of treatment; such as massage, and some surgical procedures. These are, however, used only within the framework of magico-religious therapeutics which consist of conjuring, magical charms, invocations, songs and dances. This follows naturally from the basic concept of the primitives that all illnesses are of supernatural origin. We can explain the efficacy of these measures (and they are often quite successful) only on the basis of their psychotherapeutic elements. A closer study of these treatment

---

[1] Wieschhoff, H. A., *Concepts of Abnormality among the Ibo of Nigeria*, *J. Am. Orient. Soc.* 63: 262, 1943.

rituals reveals that they involve a great deal of confession and suggestion, and are often not very different even in form from our methods of treatment.

If we dwell a little longer on ethnographic material, we are only following an old psychiatric tradition. From Benjamin Rush and J. C. Prichard to Kraepelin and A. Marie, psychiatrists have been attracted to comparative psychiatry. In recent times, too, several ethnologists, particularly in North America (where they call themselves cultural anthropologists), seem to have contributed greatly to our understanding of the nature of mental illness, its social origins, and, in particular, the relativity of its symptoms. We refer above all to the works of Ruth Benedict, E. Sapir, I. A. Hallowell and their successors.[2] Their argument briefly is as follows: we look upon certain behavioural phenomena; such as ideas of persecution, grandiose ideas, states of ecstasy, hallucinations, compulsive ideas and marked changes of facial expression and of gesture, as symptoms of mental illness. But the study of foreign cultures has shown that all these so-called symptoms can, under different circumstances, be regarded as normal, just as so-called " pathological tissues " can be normal in a different place and at a different time. For instance, ideas of persecution are normal among the Dobuans, grandiose ideas among the Kwakiutl, and hallucinations are normal among the Mohave or Takala. Ecstatic states are normal among the Siberians and the Zulus. Homosexuality is regarded as normal by many tribes who even give their transvestites a legal status, known as Berdache. The belief in taboo often leads to behaviour which we would consider to be compulsive. Conversely, people commonly considered to be abnormal by these societies, such as kind and generous individuals in Dobu, would be regarded by us as normal. We have, therefore, thought it useful to introduce into comparative psychopathology the terms autonormal and autopathological on the one hand, and heteronormal and heteropathological on the other. Autonormal and autopathological would apply to individuals regarded as normal or pathological, respectively, by their own society; heteronormal and heteropathological to those regarded as normal or pathological, respectively, by members of another society observing them.

It follows that what is psychologically normal depends to a high

---

[2] Those interested in a detailed exposition of this material, and a comprehensive bibliography, are referred to my article, " *Psychopathology, Primitive Medicine and Primitive Culture,*" *Bull. Hist. Med.* 14: 30-67, 1943; and to Ruth Benedict's most important and easily accessible work: " *Patterns of Culture.*"

degree on the attitudes of different societies. The same is true, incidentally, of crime. The criterion by which a person in any society is
judged to be mentally ill is not primarily the presence of certain unvary-
ing and universally occurring symptoms. It depends rather on whether
the affected individual is capable of some minimum of adaptation and
social functioning within his society, or whether the psychological
change has progressed to such an extent that he has become a foreign
body in his society.

The relativity of symptoms can be observed in historical as well as
in ethnological material. Henry E. Sigerist[3] pointed out many years
ago that the troubadour who appeared quite normal to his contemporaries would by us be regarded as insane. The same is true for many
other characters of the Middle Ages and of the early Renaissance,
e.g.; the ecstatic religionists, the witch hunters and the ascetic puritans.
There is little doubt that the normal man of today would have seemed
abnormal in many earlier centuries. This may be related to the fact
that the nature of mental diseases is apparently changing with the
course of time. Thus Jaspers, for instance, sees schizophrenia as the
predominant mental illness of the present day, whereas hysteria
occurred more frequently in the nineteenth and earlier centuries.

This relativity of symptoms is seen in our own society in relation to
differences of social class and status. If a poor peasant believes in the
evil eye, one can by no means assume that he is mentally ill. If the
same belief is held by a university professor, this assumption becomes
inevitable. Modes of behaviour regarded as normal in artists or
adolescents would be regarded as abnormal in average adults. In this
connection it is interesting to note that Kinsey found clear differences
in sexual behaviour and in concepts of normality in this field among the
different classes in the United States of America; despite the fact that
there are fewer psychological class differences in the United States
than in any other modern society.

It must be pointed out here that in spite of apparent similarities in
outward guise and in content, there is a fundamental difference between
the patterns of behaviour seen in primitives and those observed in the
insane. The ideas of persecution of the average Dobuan, and the
ideas of grandeur of a Kwakiutl, are not held by them as individuals,
but because each one thinks within the conceptual framework of his
culture; and because such ideas are held by the majority of their

[3] " *Psychopathologie und Kulturwissenschaft* " *Abh. aus der Neurol. Psychiatrie,
Psychol. u. ihren Grenzgeb.* Vol. 61, p. 140-146, 1930.

tribes. The exceptional individual, who in our culture is the victim of ideas of grandeur or of persecution, does not thereby share the concepts of his culture. On the contrary, he is unable to make these concepts his own. This point should also be remembered when comparing the often apparently very similar artistic productions of the insane and of children on the one hand, with those of primitives on the other.

This is not, of course, to deny the possibility that behind this multiplicity of symptoms there may lie in all societies the same biological disposition to disease—an absolute abnormality per se. The difficulty is, of course, that we have no absolute biological criteria for diagnosing or classifying even the most widespread psychoses and neuroses and are, therefore, forced to rely largely on their symptomatology, and on their effect on the patient's capacity to conform to the society in which he lives. This difficulty is not lessened, as far as comparative pathology is concerned, by the fact that psychoses known to have an organic basis, such as general paresis, alcoholism, and senile dementia, do not exist among the savages.

The relativity of symptoms is by no means limited to the field of mental diseases. In somatic medicine also it is often not the absolute state of affairs but society's evaluation of it which decides whether a biological variation is to be regarded as a disease or not. It did not occur to the Chinese of classical times to look upon the crippled feet of their women as signs of illness. Many African tribes do not regard infestation with intestinal worms or yaws as illnesses, probably because they are so common. It is reported, somewhat grotesquely, that among some South American Indians a very disfiguring spirochaetal infection of the skin, known as pinto, is so widespread that almost all men suffer from it. The few who escape infection are regarded as ill and are precluded from marriage. It has been shown historically that malaria was so prevalent in many parts of the world in the nineteenth century (e.g. in the Mississippi Valley), that it was no longer regarded as a disease. The same was true for eczema among children in the eighteenth century.

If we must assume, therefore, that the prevalence and definition of mental disease depend upon social circumstances, it follows that mental illnesses must vary in form and magnitude in different tribes, cultures and civilizations. This is indeed the case. There are, however, no tribes in which all members are insane, nor are there tribes in which mental illness or suicide are unknown. The latter, once a widespread assumption, is merely a vestige of Rousseau's illusion of the " noble savage."

Hallowell, on the contrary, has rightly pointed out that ideas about supernatural forces can at times have beneficial and healing effects on mental illnesses; but can also result in pathogenic fears and conflicts. In addition, it must not be forgotten that most of the so-called savages are, or were, observed, not in their " natural state " but in a state of " acculturation," as it is called in North America; that is, at a moment in their history in which their own culture was threatened both physically and psychologically by a foreign culture. This state appears to encourage the development of individual and of collective psychoses.

Although, therefore, mental illness appears to exist everywhere, many serious observers have pointed out that some forms of mental illness common in our culture, for example schizophrenia, are not found in such diverse parts of the world as Melanesia, Brazil, Central Africa or among the North American Indians. The attempt, which has recently once again become fashionable, to force a variety of different mental illnesses into the category of schizophrenia is essentially artificial. We have already mentioned that certain organic psychoses are not found among primitives, partly because of their short life span. On the other hand, serious observers have pointed out the prevalence of mental illnesses among some primitives, e.g., among the Siberian tribes. On the whole, however, our material is too meagre, both in quantity and in quality, to enable us to go beyond such generalisations. In some tribes it may well be possible that mental illnesses are rare because of favourable conditions. In others it may be that psychotherapy is effective, or that the sick are killed outright.[4] It is also possible that psychiatrically untrained visitors may, in the absence of a local distinction between mental and physical diseases, often have overlooked endemic forms of mental illnesses and may have described some as physical illnesses. We possess only a single statistical example in this whole field; and even this is of doubtful value in several respects. N. Skliar and K. Starikova (*Zur vergleichenden Psychiatrie: Arch. f. Psychiatrie und Nervenkrankheiten*, 88: 554-85, 1929) compared the incidence of mental illnesses among seven national groups in the province of Astrakhan. Two of the groups, the Kalmucks and the Kirghiz, remained quite primitive for a considerable period of time. The results were as follows:

(1) The incidence of mental illness was very low amongst these tribes at the beginning of the period reported on: in fact it was

almost non-existent. Kalmucks 1850: 0.01%. Kirghiz hospital admission rate 1890: 0.4 per 100,000.

(2) Contact with civilization, such as occurred after 1850, was accompanied by a steady rise in the figures (Kalmucks 1898: 0.07%. Kirghiz hospital admission rates 1927: 3.0 per 100,000). The greater the distance between a Kalmuck tribe and the civilised areas, the lower were the figures. The incidence of mental diseases in both tribes was far lower than that of the neighbouring, civilized communities (Kalmucks 2-14 per 100,000; Tartars 3-60; Armenians 90; Jews 50; Russians and Persians 100 per 100,000). The influence of civilization was not attributable to alcohol or syphilis. In both tribes syphilis was endemic but general paresis did not occur. The Kalmuck tribe had always been alcoholic: the moslem Kirghiz continued to be abstinent.

(3) Dementia praecox continued to be rare among the primitives (Kalmucks 2.6% of all mental illnesses; Kirghiz 1.9%, compared with 6.4% among the Russians and 20% among the Armenians). Neither hysteria nor general paresis was observed among these tribes.

(4) Whilst these tendencies were found in both tribes, they differed considerably with respect to their prevalence among men and women. Among the Kalmucks there were twice as many women mentally ill as men; among the Kirghiz suffering from mental illness the sex ratio reached the unusually high figure of eight men to one woman. Between 1890 and 1902, five to thirty times as many Kalmucks were admitted to hospital as were Kirghiz. In 1925 to 1927 these figures were three to ten.

It is worth noting that some forms of mental illness which occur in primitive peoples are difficult or impossible to fit into our own categories of disease. There is first of all Amuck; the familiar murderous psychosis, first observed among the Malay, but later also among South American Indians, Melanesians, Siberians, Indians and also the Masai. A neurosis characterised above all by echolalia and echopraxia was first observed in Siberia and was described in climatic terms as Arctic hysteria; until it was found to occur frequently in East India, in the Philippines and in Madagascar. It is now generally referred to by the Malay name of "Latah." Imu, a disease of the Ainu, is a strange combination of Latah and Amuck. A cannibalistic psychosis of North American Indians, in some ways reminiscent of the "Vaudoisie" of the fifteenth century,[5] has become known as " Windigo." Certain intoxicants, such as Indian hemp, also, of course, evoke special psychoses. It is noteworthy that alcoholism can have different manifestations in different tribes. Perhaps the most remarkable of the psychoses observed among primitive people is that known as Thanatomania, or death by autosuggestion, in which the patient believes he has been bewitched, and dies without visible organic changes. This has been described and studied under the name " Voodoo death " by the famous physiologist, W. B. Cannon.[6] In all these cases it is obvious that the nature of the illness is determined not by climate nor by racial factors, but by the culture; that is, by the sum total of social relationships. Much has been written about mass psychoses among primitive people. But, as Griesinger has already pointed out, one must be careful to avoid misinterpreting purely religious movements as mass phychoses.

These ethnological considerations would be incomplete without some mention of the medicine man; the physician of the primitives, who is, in many books, still referred to as an epileptic, an hysteric, a neurotic, and even as an idiot. Such descriptions appear to be completely false and to be due to ignorance or misunderstanding. They are refuted by all present-day ethnologists who have had personal experience among savages. It is true that in a few parts of the world (particularly in Siberia and South-east Africa) individuals who are known to have experienced a psychosis later turn to the art of healing. But at the time of practising their profession, and perhaps because of their choice of profession, they are healthy; in the sense of being fully able to perform their social functions. Individuals who are suffering from a real mental disease are rejected as physicians by the natives themselves. The Siberian name of " Shaman " should be reserved for these individuals and not used indiscriminately for all medicine men. A further group of native practitioners appeared to previous untrained European observers to be pathological, since they developed trance states and were possessed by helpful spirits. Such states, however, are autonormal in these tribes; are distinguished by the natives themselves from possession by evil spirits, that is, from hysterical or epileptic attacks; are regarded as desirable, and are, therefore, in some measure encouraged. The great majority of medicine men seem to be normal even by our criteria. In fact, many trained ethnologists; such as Elkin, Hallowell, Olbrecht, Warner, Seligman, Stoll and Shiroko-

---

[5] Cesbron, H., *Histoire Critique de l'Hystérie*, Paris, 1909, p. 134.
[6] Cannon, W. B., *Voodoo Death.*, *Am. Anthropologist*, 44: 169, 1942.

goroff; have emphasised their superior intelligence and complete normality, despite their ideas which we find so strange.

The assumption that medicine men or savages who believe in magic are mentally ill, is only a special instance of the bad habit, so widespread in our society, of dismissing as psychopathological everything that is different and not at once open to our understanding. " The undefinable is regarded as psychopathic."

It seemed for a time as if psychiatry and ethnology[7] would continue to benefit from each other; for example, when Malinowski showed that among the Trobrianders the so-called " Oedipus complex " was not directed against the father, but against the authority figure of the mother's brother. But unfortunately most of the ethnologists who are interested in psychiatry have accepted with naïve gullibility the tenets of psychoanalysis or one of its derivative schools; so that their later works are full of fantasy rather than fact.

Psychiatry itself has for some time recognised that psychological illnesses are socially determined, and the move away from an absolutism of symptoms began some hundred years ago. It cannot be denied, however, that in both directions the study of ethnographic material has been, and will continue to be, of great value.

---

[7] The reader is referred to the following comprehensive expositions of the more recent relationships between ethnology and psychiatry: Kluckhohn, C. *The Influence of Psychiatry on Anthropology in America*, in " *Hundred Years of American Psychiatry*," New York, 1944, p. 589; Caudill, W., *Applied Anthropology in Medicine*, in " *Anthropology Today*," A. L. Kroeber ed. Chicago, 1953; Opler, M. R., *Culture, Psychiatry and Human Values*, Springfield, 1956.

CHAPTER II

GRECO-ROMAN PSYCHIATRY

THE history of psychiatry, like that of scientific medicine in general, really begins with the Greeks. The Greco-Roman outlook survived unchanged until the eighteenth century, and even today we still use a large part of the Greek nomenclature. While the great cultures of old, such as those of Egypt and Mesopotamia, vacillated between naturalistic and supernatural explanations of diseases, the Greeks declared themselves outspokenly in favour of naturalistic explanations and thus became the founders of scientific medicine and of psychiatry. This applies, of course, only to the Greek medical profession. In other spheres religious concepts continued to survive, and religious explanations of disease and methods of treatment were at least as common outside official medical practice in the Greek culture as in our own.

The introductory remarks to the Hippocratic book on epilepsy, the " sacred disease," are typical of the new outlook: " The position regarding the so-called sacred disease is as follows: It seems to me to be no more divine and no more sacred than other diseases, but, like other affections, it springs from natural causes . . . Those who first connected this illness with demons and described it as sacred seem to me no different from the conjurors, purificators, mountebanks and charlatans of our day, who pretend to great piety and superior knowledge. But such persons are merely concealing, under the cloak of godliness, their perplexity and their inability to afford any assistance." (Grimm, J. F. C., *The Works of Hippocrates*, Glogau, 1838, Vol. 2, p. 211). In this way those formerly regarded as being possessed were now thought to be ill, and, according to the Greek ideas about illness, to be physically ill. Greek medicine, like primitive medicine, is monistic, only on a new and completely different basis.

Unfortunately for us, there is a great poverty of Greco-Roman documents relating to mental illnesses. It is hard to say whether this is attributable to the loss of manuscripts or to a lack of interest in these diseases. Such material as does exist comes from the later period of antiquity; but it can no longer be assumed, as was done in the past, that this necessarily reflects an increase during that later period in the incidence of mental disorder. The two giants of Greek medicine, Hippocrates and Galen, have left behind only occasional accounts relating to mental illnesses. Pinel blamed Galen for his lack of interest in psychiatry, which he said was the reason for the lack of progress in this field until the eighteenth century. Our main sources are: Celsus (*circa* 30 A.D.), the Roman encyclopaedist, who in his book: " *De re medica*," presents us with a chapter on the treatment of melancholia and of mania; and Aretaeus of Cappadocia (*circa* 150 A.D.) in whose book: " *Acute and Chronic Disease*," we find short chapters on the nature of melancholia and mania and on the treatment of phrenitis and melancholia. Our best source is the methodist, Soranus of Ephesus (*circa* 100 A.D.), whose two major works on acute and on chronic diseases have survived in a Latin translation of Caelius Aurelianus (*circa* 500 A.D.); of which there is an excellent English translation and edition by I. E. Drabkin (Chicago, 1950). The work on acute diseases contains several chapters on phrenitis and its treatment. That on chronic diseases contains chapters on mania and melancholia and their treatment. It is characteristic of the period that none of these authors wrote separate books on mental diseases, but incorporated their discussions of them in general medical works.

Greek medicine experienced many changes in the thousand years of its independent existence and produced many different points of view. Soranus himself was the adherent of only one of these; Methodism. His concepts, however, of the basic patterns of mental diseases are so similar to those of the other writers of the time that the best and easiest way of gaining some knowledge of Greek psychiatry is to begin with a summary of his ideas:[1]

According to Soranus, phrenitis is so called because the mind (*phren*, originally the diaphragm); that is, thinking, is affected. Soranus

---

[1] The "classical" theory of disease, as is well known (that of Hippocrates and Galen), is the theory of the four humours. The body consists of four different juices: blood, yellow bile, black bile, and phlegm, which correspond to the four elements: air, fire, earth and water. To each humour belong two of the four qualities: hot, moist, dry and cold. One humour predominates in each of the four temperaments: the sanguine, choleric, melancholic and phlegmatic. All diseases are caused by a disturbance of equilibrium of the humours, by the predominance or failure of one of them. Melancholia, for example, is a disease caused by the hypothetical black bile. After 300 B.C., however, other schools and factions came into being in Greek medicine, and these developed a solidist pathology and attributed diseases to changes in the solid components of the body. The best known of these schools was Methodism, which regarded all illnesses as being caused by an abnormal constriction or relaxation of the body tissues (*status strictus* and *status laxus*).

begins with a critical review of the definitions of phrenitis given by Herophilus and by Asclepiades and then presents his own definition: an acute disease of the mind accompanied by acute fever, foolish gesticulations and a small, full pulse. We are thus obviously dealing with febrile delirium. Soranus then discusses, in a typically Greek manner and with much clinical detail, the arguments for and against the existence of prodromal signs of phrenitis such as insomnia, polyuria, headache, injected eyes, etc. He believes that there is no single specific sign, but that one can predict the onset of this illness, which he regards as a very serious one, from a combination of such symptoms. He then turns to consider the differential diagnosis of phrenitis, mania, melancholia, pleurisy, pneumonia and mandrake and henbane poisoning. He asks how one can differentiate mania accompanied by fever from phrenitis, and how one can distinguish healthy sleep occurring during the course of phrenitis from the development of lethargy (coma) in this condition. Among other signs, the colour and expression of the face, respiration, pulse, stance and body temperature should be taken into account.

He then turns to more theoretical considerations. As a methodist, he rejects as merely symptomatic the subdivision of phrenitis into gay and sad forms. He suggests instead a subdivision into phrenitis on the basis of status strictus (tension) and phrenitis occurring on the basis of status laxus (relaxation). Some writers, he says, look for the seat of phrenitis in the brain, others in the head or in the aorta. Each in fact looks for it in the place which he believes to be the seat of the soul. Soranus himself regards phrenitis as a general disease but admits that, on the basis of the symptoms, the head seems to be the part most seriously affected, and should therefore be the focus of attention.

In the treatment of phrenitis, Soranus recommends isolation in a moderately light, warm and airy room, with high windows so that the patient cannot jump out. The following is characteristic of his undogmatic attitude: according to theory, phrenitis due to tension should be nursed in a well-lit room, whilst phrenitis due to exhaustion should be nursed in a dark room. But Soranus declares that if a patient reacts differently, then one should treat him in the manner which best suits his inclinations. In status strictus he must be kept awake. The attendants should enter into a few of his delusions, but should reject others. If insufficient attendants are available, the patient should be carefully fettered in order to keep him quiet. Soranus recommends warm poultices of oil, to be applied particularly to the head, and also careful blood-letting. On the third or fourth day the head should be shaved and treated with cupping, leeches and scarification. Passive exercises such as rocking, and a careful diet, are indicated. Wine should not be allowed.

One should maintain a serious attitude towards abnormally cheerful patients and a friendly one towards those who are downcast. Excitement which can evoke physical illness even in healthy people is to be avoided; since there is very great danger that it might precipitate a relapse.

Soranus then deals in a polemic manner with the treatment methods advocated by other writers such as Diocles, Erasistratus, Heraclides, and especially Asclepiades, which differ from his own in certain details. When a state of stupor follows on phrenitis, he calls it lethargy. He uses the term catalepsy to denote stupor accompanied by fever. His description of catalepsy could fit that of meningitis. He then goes on to describe other acute illnesses such as pleurisy, pneumonia, apoplexy, ileus, tetanus, etc.

In his chapter on mania or insanity or raving madness, he reports that Plato recognised two forms of mania; one of divine origin and one due to physical exertion. He concerns himself only with the latter. His definition is: a disturbance of reason without fever. Mania is found most commonly in young men and least often in women and children. Some of the causes are latent. The demonstrable causes are over-exertion, licentiousness, alcoholism and a lack of discharge such as is brought about by bleeding from haemorrhoids or by menstruation.

This theory was maintained in all seriousness until the nineteenth century. Mania, according to Soranus, had the same prodromata as had epilepsy and apoplexy. It could occur continuously or in intermittent attacks. Its manifestations were fury, gaiety, sadness, silliness or anxiety, such as, for example, a persistent fear of falling into ditches. Some patients were unable to visit underground chambers on account of this fear. Patients in these deluded states may see themselves as sparrows, cockerels, earthenware vessels, gods, orators, actors, grains of corn, the centre of the universe, or as infants. The eyes are injected, the body is firm and abnormally strong. The symptoms suggest that mania is a physical disease affecting in particular the head, and is due to status strictus. Soranus rejects the view of the philosophers that mania is a disease of the soul (diaphysis) and attributes their therapeutic failures to their misconceptions. It will be remembered that Plato, in his *Charmides*, had paid a similar compliment to the physicians of his day when he accused them of inability either to understand or to cure mental diseases.

The description of the treatment of mania is basically similar to that of phrenitis, and therefore need not be repeated. Soranus makes a few minor additions, such as listening to dripping water in cases of insomnia, massage, and going for walks. He further recommends strengthening the patients' reasoning powers by asking them questions, or getting them to read and criticize texts which contain false statements. Apart from this, the patients should spend their time in light reading, play acting (the plays should be in a spirit contrary to the patients' mental states), or delivering speeches to a friendly audience. The tasks allotted to patients should be selected according to their previous education. Chess and travel are also recommended. These methods in large measure can be traced back at least to Asclepiades (c. 100 B.C.). The patient should be treated energetically in the acute stages of the illness, gently during remissions. Soranus makes use of hellebore as an emetic. However, he rejects a large number of therapeutic measures; among them darkness, starvation, continuous fettering, opium, excessive blood-letting, enemata, alcohol, whipping, music and love.

The chapter on melancholia is appreciably shorter. Soranus is a methodist and believes in a solidist pathology. He does not, therefore, see melancholia as black bile, but as " black rage." He considers that it occurs most commonly in men at the prime of life, and that it can be caused by digestive upsets, drugs, fear and grief. The main symptoms are depression, mutism, death wishes, marked suspiciousness, weeping, muttering and occasional joviality. Melancholia is not a form of mania. The latter is a disease of the head, while melancholia is a disease of the oesophagus. Treatment is the same as for mania, except that local measures should be directed not at the head but at the regions of the stomach and shoulder blades. Soranus advises against the use of hellebore, blood-letting and excessively powerful drugs.

Summarising his views and comparing them with those of others, we can say that Soranus, like Celsus and Aretaeus, recognised three main mental diseases: phrenitis, mania and melancholia. He did not even mention hysteria, which was described by Aretaeus. It should be noted that on one occasion the latter mentioned senile dementia in passing. All three writers were extreme somaticists. The body-soul dualism which predominated among Greek philosophers was to them an alien concept. Their analysis and general treatment of the three mental diseases is based on the assumption that they are dealing with physical illnesses. Only homosexuality is regarded by Soranus as an illness of the psyche. Aretaeus thought that hysteria was a disease of the uterus (wandering of the uterus), and went so far as to deal with it alongside fatal uterine haemorrhages and inflammations. Despite this, he recognised that the same disease picture could occur in men. In him, also, clinical observation triumphed over theoretical considerations.

Although mental diseases were regarded as physical illnesses, the brain was rarely mentioned. This is not surprising, since the ancient Greeks were grossly deficient in their concepts both of the functions of this organ and of the peripheral nerves. The emphasis put on phrenitis may have been partly a subjective one and partly due to the predominance of febrile illnesses, or to misdiagnosis, since fever was diagnosed only by hand. Aretaeus, incidentally, pointed out the interesting difference that while in phrenitis perception itself was disturbed, in melancholia and mania what was perceived was wrongly interpreted.

Neither mania nor melancholia can be recognised in any of our present-day syndromes. Mania simply meant an agitated form of insanity; melancholia a quiet one. Aretaeus's view that melancholia may pass into mania can, therefore, only with some qualifications be regarded as foreshadowing manic-depressive psychosis. His theory that melancholia was generally limited to a single " phantasy " was frequently put forward in later years.

In contrast to Greek tradition in general, Soranus did not discuss prognosis in mental diseases. Aretaeus, however, stressed the frequency of relapses, and the fact that these illnesses were, in practice, often of lifelong duration and that they frequently terminated in states of silliness or of paralysis (!) Because mental illnesses were often incurable, the physician was thought to have the moral right to refuse to undertake treatment. This right, incidentally, was accorded to the medical profession until the end of the eighteenth century.

Soranus's treatment consisted essentially of isolation, moderate blood-letting, diet, massage, and local treatments applied to the head and the oesophagus. In complete contrast to his basic assumptions, he also made use of psychotherapy. Celsus and Aretaeus held very different theories about the nature of mental illness and the seat of the soul. Their descriptions, however, of these diseases and their treatment closely resembled those of Soranus; with the difference that as humoral pathologists, they laid greater stress on blood-letting and the use of cathartics and drugs in general. Celsus was also a great deal more ruthless. His " psychotherapy " includes measures such as menaces, torture, whipping, and sudden, brutal ducking.

Greek psychiatry presents us with the first clinical observations and with the first attempts at a classification of mental illnesses. It was never a slave to its own theories. Treatment was essentially physical, sometimes psychological, and always empirical. Although its successes did not measure up to those in other branches of Greek medicine, it is still of considerable importance, particularly when one considers subsequent achievements in psychiatry.

CHAPTER III

RENAISSANCE PSYCHIATRY

THERE is almost nothing to say about mediaeval psychiatry, because we know very little about mediaeval medicine, and because, in contrast to achievements in other spheres, little of positive value emerged in the field of medicine during the Middle Ages. On the contrary, much occurred that was harmful. The worst was probably the disintegration of medicine. Surgery fell into the hands of barbers and their assistants, psychiatry into the hands of exorcising priests and clerical witch hunters. Individual physicians attempted, with greater or lesser success, to maintain the Greek traditions; as Temkin has demonstrated so well in the special case of epilepsy.[1] The naturalistic ideas of the ancients about mental diseases must, therefore, have survived in certain places and among certain strata of society. Hospitals for the insane were built: (Metz, 1100; Braunschweig, 1224; Bedlam, 1377), above all, by the Arabs: (Fez, *circa* 700; Bagdad, 705; Cairo, 800; Damascus and Aleppo, 1270). These kept alive the scientific ideas of the Greeks about insanity. Occasional attempts were even made to develop these further; as for example by Najab, who is said to have described nine groups of mental illnesses with thirty sub-groups.

On the whole, however, what little knowledge the Greeks had established was lost, and a tragic decline to an earlier cultural level ensued. The clock was put back by a thousand years. For over a thousand years the mentally ill were again regarded as possessed by the devil and by evil spirits, or were considered to be witches or sorcerers who could produce the illness in others. " Apparitions " and hallucinations were thought of as the work of the devil. The result was, of course, that the physician was excluded from the field of mental illnesses, the study of which was taken over by the Inquisitors. In the Middle Ages one does not find observations about the mentally ill in medical text books,

---

[1] Temkin, O., *The Falling Sickness*, Baltimore, 1945. Whitwell, J. R., *Historical Notes on Psychiatry*, London, 1936, contains translations of several mediaeval physicians. See also Wright, E. H., *Mediaeval Attitudes towards Mental Sickness*, *Bull. Hist. Med.* 7: 352, 1939.

but rather in the handbooks and protocols of the witch hunters and exorcists. From the psychiatric point of view the Middle Ages are also notable for the frequency of psychic epidemics or mass psychoses; such as the flagellationist movement, dancing mania, childrens' crusades, persecution of the Jews and " possession " of total communities of people, particularly in monasteries.[2] On the other hand, one must not overlook the fact that some mediaeval institutions, such as the monasteries or pilgrimages, often served as a refuge and source of help for psychologically sick people.

The degradation of psychiatry by no means came to an end during the brilliant period of the Renaissance and the onset of the modern age. On the contrary, it was at this time that the lunacy of the sane reached its climax. During the whole of the Middle Ages, although many devils were exorcised, the number of witches executed was probably nowhere near the number burned at the stake during the relatively enlightened fifteenth century and the subsequent two hundred years. The *Malleus Maleficarum*, the infamous handbook of the witch hunters, which was written by the Dominicans Heinrich Kraemer and Jakob Sprenger, appeared as late as 1486. It shows clearly that not only the possessed but also a large number of witches were in fact mentally ill. The most renowned physicians of the Renaissance; men such as Fernel, Paré and Johannes Lange, were among the most ardent believers in this barbarous nonsense.[3]

A small elite of outstanding medical men, however, emerged during the Renaissance who made new and honourable contributions to psychiatry. They declared that many possessed and many witches had nothing whatever to do with the devil or with other supernatural forces, but had become mentally ill for very natural reasons, and merited medical attention and not the stake. They thus publicly expressed opinions which, according to the polemics of the *Malleus Maleficarum*, had been whispered among the " Heretics." Although the words and deeds of Cornelius Agrippa, Della Porta, Cardano, Paracelsus, Lemnius, Reginald Scotus and Johann Weyer still show many mediaeval traits, they are fully worthy of the high-sounding title, given them by Zilboorg, of " The first psychiatric revolution." Other men, like Gesner,

---

[2] Calmeil, L. F., *De la folie considerée sous le rapport pathologique, historique et judiciaire*, Paris, 1845.

[3] In order to avoid misplaced optimism, it is unfortunately necessary to point out that similar irrational and paranoid ideas can be found even in the twentieth century, although here they usually appear in the guise of " naturalism " rather than of the supernatural.

Montanus, Benedictus and Schenck von Grafenberg, reported cases of mental disease and their treatment by natural means, without discussing " possession " as such.

Both the increase of witch hunting and the beginning of the scientific protest are aspects of the Renaissance which can probably be attributed to the same basic phenomenon; namely the moral-ideological and politico-economic disintegration of mediaeval society. This stimulated and encouraged a few great minds towards an increased freedom of thought, but filled the majority with panic and anxiety. It provoked the upholders of the old system to irrational counter-attacks on the devil and his handymen, and the almost unendurable celibacy of the Inquisitors added the particular misogynous flavour to this movement. On the basis of the *Malleus Maleficarum*, everyone who showed the slightest psychological deviation or peculiarity was regarded as a witch or a sorcerer. Not only mental diseases but almost all afflictions of the body (impotence, sterility, deformity, death in infancy), and all misfortunes of life (a poor harvest, death, a broken marriage), were attributed to the works of the devil and his servants.

One must, however, avoid misconceptions about the modernism of the men responsible for the psychiatric revolution. They too were the children of their time and advanced not by leaps and bounds, but one step at a time. Even this, however, was enough to draw upon them both the hatred and persecution of their contemporaries and to earn them the gratitude and admiration of later generations. Among the products of the new " psychiatry," the one which aroused the greatest enmity was the book by Johann Weyer of Brabant (1515-1588), " *De Praestigiis Daemonum*," which appeared in 1563. Weyer[4] begins with a description of the devil, his attributes and his cohorts. The power of the devil, like that of witches is, he says, limited by God, and as a non-corporeal being the devil is unable to engage in many activities with which he has been credited, such as, for example, sexual intercourse. Weyer remarks that natural events are often regarded as works of the devil. He believes not only in the devil, but also in so-called evil magicians, such as Arnald of Villanova, Roger Bacon and Faust. He demands their punishment and excepts only his teacher, Cornelius Agrippa, who, according to Weyer, did not belong to their group.

Next he turns to witches. It appears obvious to him that the activities

---

[4] Johann Weyer (Wierus): born 1515 in Grave, North Brabant; studied in Bonn, Paris and Orleans; 1545, city medical officer of Arnheim; 1550-1578, private physician to Duke William of Julich-Cleve-Berg; died 1588.

described by witches are not real (and therefore not punishable), but are fancies given to them by the devil. The devil's work is made easy in their case; since witches are usually people suffering from melancholic mental illnesses, and patients so afflicted are known to be already predisposed to disturbance of the imagination. Furthermore, it would be blasphemous to regard the activities of witches as real, because one would then be attributing to them and to the devil deeds which God alone can perform. Occasionally the phantasies of witches can be traced to the use of belladonna ointments, and here Weyer refers to the experiments of Della Porta and Cardano with such ointments. Magic, he says, is not, in fact, efficacious and it would be better to treat witches with sympathy. The tests to which they are submitted are senseless. The foreign bodies, such as nails, knives, etc., which they vomit up are not their own productions but have been introduced in them by the devil by means of sorcery. Sometimes these objects can have a natural origin. Impotence, he says, is due to natural causes. Lycanthropy (the belief of having been changed into a wolf), is not due to witchcraft but to madness. Somewhere else, however, Weyer states that this is an illusion attributable to the work of the devil. The possessed are either mentally ill people suffering from melancholia, or charlatans with a great desire to feel important. Weyer was particularly clever at exposing such frauds.

In the treatment of the possessed, he says, the priests have turned religion into magic. Their methods of treatment are successful because they act on the imagination. In cases of possession a doctor should be called in first. His purges can sometimes be beneficial, even in the case of illness due to supernatural causes. Subsequently one should send the patient to a priest for a kind of re-education.

These, briefly, are the opinions defended by Weyer in his " De Praestigiis Daemonum." They are a mixture of traditional views, theological criticism and original clinical observations. In other fields also Weyer was a very able clinician. I think it would be a mistake to assume, as has so often been done, that Weyer was hypocritical and in fact no longer believed in any supernatural causes for disease. There is no evidence for this. On the contrary, it is much more likely and more natural that Weyer still believed in the devil and in evil magicians. But that is not the most important part of his work. The important part is that he recognised the witches and the possessed as mentally ill and demanded that they should primarily be treated by the doctor and not by the priest. Weyer is neither the first nor the only representative of such views. He himself had heard them from his teacher, Cornelius Agrippa, and could find them in the writings of Della Porta, Cardano, Andrea a Laguna, Amatus Lusitanus and Paracelsus. But he was their most explicit, most forceful and most successful champion.

The Renaissance is an age of deep contradictions. Side by side with the ruthless persecution of the insane as witches, we find everywhere signs of a deep sympathy for those suffering from these diseases. This diversity of attitudes found expression not only in the writings of the authors already cited, but also in the setting up of numerous institutions for the insane. This occurred particularly in Spain, which at that time experienced a " golden era " of medicine and of civilization in general, and where Arabian influences were most strongly felt. Institutions for the mentally ill were built in Seville in 1409, in Saragossa and Valencia in 1410, in Barcelona in 1412 and in Toledo in 1483. It is typical of the age that some few decades later the repentant veteran soldier, Bernadino Alvarez, built a similar institution in newly conquered Mexico (San Hippolyto); the first of its kind in the American continent. The writings of the Spanish humanist, Juan Luis Vives (1492-1540), also vividly express this sympathetic understanding for the mentally ill.

The significance of the Renaissance for psychiatry, however, goes beyond the rebirth of a humane attitude towards the insane. Doubts as to the supernatural causation of mental illness and other phenomena, such as miracles, which had previously been explained on this basis, led to a search for natural forces and natural causes; and we now find the concept of " imaginatio," for example, in the writings of the above-mentioned authors, as well as in those of Pomponatius, Libavius and Pico della Mirandola. This imaginatio is very similar to our present-day concept of suggestion. It is a force capable of causing both physical and psychological illnesses and also of curing them. Since we ourselves are not very clear as to what exactly we mean by suggestion, we should not be too critical of the sixteenth century workers if they also remain somewhat vague as to the exact nature of their imaginatio.

Whatever one's opinion of Paracelsus,[5] he was undoubtedly the most renowned physician of his time, and for this reason alone he

---

[5] Philippus Aureolus Theophratus Bombastus von Hohenheim, called Paracelsus: Born 1491 in Maria Einsiedeln, son of a doctor. 1502, moved with his father to Villach in Carinthia, Austria, seat of the mines of the Fugger family. Early contact there with alchemy. From 1507, wandering scholar; Tuebingen, Heidelberg, Freiburg, Cologne, Erfurt, Vienna. 1513, Ferrara, where he is said to have taken a degree. Army surgeon in Italy, Holland, Sweden. Also travelled

would merit our attention. He was, in addition, more concerned with psychiatry than were his contemporaries. About 1520, he wrote a small book called " *Diseases which lead to a Loss of Reason*," which was published in 1567. In his introductory remarks he makes it quite clear that whatever the clerics might say, mental illnesses are not caused by spirits, but are natural diseases. This was a courageous and extremely valuable statement to make in his day. Although his writings abound in Greek, Roman and Arabic ideas, Paracelsus was concerned to build up a new system of medicine, and he created a new classification of mental diseases in place of the classical triad of mania, melancholia and phrenitis. He distinguished the following mental illnesses: epilepsy, mania, " true insanity," St. Vitus dance and suffocatio intellectus (the old hysteria).

He described five types of epilepsy; arising from the brain, the liver, the heart, the intestines and the limbs. This was not an unusual concept for his time. His clinical description (fainting, seizures, sudden or gradual falling, frothing and occasionally incontinence of urine) shows that he did not clearly differentiate between epilepsy and hysteria. Epilepsy, according to him, could occur in any living thing, not only in lions and squirrels, but also in trees. It was a disturbance of the spiritus vitae, precipitated by food or " vapours." In accord with his philosophy of the macrocosmos-microcosmos, he likened it to an earthquake. The illness, he said, began as early as intra-uterine life and consisted, first and foremost, of seething of the spiritus vitae in the various organs of its origin.

Mania, he said, consisted of a disturbance of reason and not of the senses. Its manifestations were excited and unreasonable behaviour, agitation and irritability. There was a tendency to relapse, and the illness could be primary; occurring in physically healthy persons, or it could be secondary to other diseases. A substance whose vapours rose to the brain was distilled either above or below the diaphragm. If this substance originated from excreta, the patients would refuse food, would talk to themselves, would be given to vomiting and would ignore their surroundings. If it were distilled in the limbs, they would be cheerful, wild and excited. If the temperature were high, the humor vitae would burn, its finer particles would be separated

in Spain, Portugal, France, England, Russia, Turkey, Egypt and the Balkans. 1524, attempted to settle in Salzburg but failed because of the peasant wars. 1526, Professor at Basle, but 1528 had to flee from there. Continued a life of wandering in Southern Germany, Switzerland, Bohemia and Austria. 1532, religious crisis. Died in Salzburg, 1541.

off and would rise upwards. The substance at times coagulated in the head and might change into worms; at other times it would lead to the formation of ulcers. The spontaneous generation of worms was not questioned until at least the seventeenth century. Paracelsus naturally disputed the theory of the four temperaments and the four humours. Mania, he said, arose from the spiritus vitae alone. It uncovered secret " attitudes and qualities " in the afflicted persons which, until then, had been latent.

True insanity (" those who are really mad ") he described as a permanent state related to the stars. He distinguished five sub-groups: lunatici, insani, vesani, melancholici and obsessi. The first four, he said, had nothing to do with the devil, for where there is no reason, the devil has lost his rights. Such patients do not suffer pain as do those afflicted with mania, chorea lasciva, suffocatio intellectus or epilepsy. In the case of lunatici, the spiritus vitae is under the invisible influence of the moon and the stars; just as iron is influenced by a magnet, or as water is drawn from the earth by the sun. The insani are born mad (this was a new point of view), either because the semen was diseased, or because they were affected by the moon in utero. The vesani are poisoned with food or drink, particularly with food which has been subjected to the magic of love. Some patients think of nothing but love, some only of war, and yet others of climbing and running.

" St. Vitus dance " (dancing mania) could not, according to him, be attributed to the saints, since these do not cause diseases. He suggested chorea lasciva as a more appropriate name for it and said it was due either to the precipitation of certain irritating salts in the veins of laughter by the spiritus vitae, or to imaginatio (imagination and imitation).

His suffocatio intellectus again appears to be a combination of epilepsy and hysteria. He described it as a natural disease due either to intestinal worms, intra-uterine events, over-eating or excessive sleeping. Intestinal worms were still regarded as the main cause of mental illnesses by the well known Paris pathologist, Prost, at the beginning of the nineteenth century. Again, according to Paracelsus, the illness was due to fumes from the affected organs reaching the head or being sucked into the heart. Pressure in these organs could cause tremors, seizures and sometimes death. The illnesses could also be precipitated by blows to the head. Paracelsus mentions head injuries so frequently as a cause of seizures and insanity that one can regard him as a forerunner of J. H. Jackson.

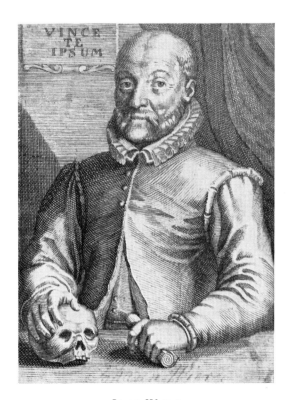

JOHN WEYER

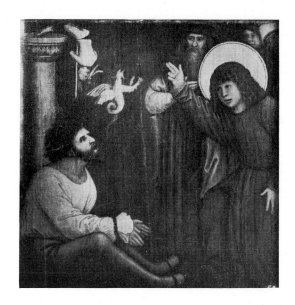

St. Vitus cures possession
(Swabian painting XIIth century)

Only brief mention will be made of the chapters on therapy in Paracelsus's " *Diseases which lead to a Loss of Reason.*" They are remarkable for the absence of any mention of psychotherapy and for their emphasis on chemical measures. In the case of epilepsy, Paracelsus departs from his basic rule that physical diseases should be treated only by physical drugs, and " spiritual " diseases only by " spiritual " drugs. For the " spiritual " affliction of epilepsy he prescribed such physical means as camphor, powdered unicorn, etc. He then lists a number of " spiritual " drugs whose effect was coagulating, astringent or specific. All illnesses were, he said, curable with his Arcana, which were manufactured not by the physicians but by the " artists " (the alchemists). Some of his recipes for Arcana, like Hungarian vitriol or oil of Arcani, contain camphor, skull shavings, unicorn, herbs and root plants. In the treatment of mania one should allow the vapours to escape by opening primarily those parts of the body to which mania rises (toes, fingers, head). He also recommends cooling and astringent measures to combat the dangerous vapours. In the case of lunatici, it was important to counteract the magnetic attracting forces of the moon or the sun by certain means such as his so-called quintessences; especially the " quinta essentia auri." Congenital madness should be prevented by means of " coitus artificialis " between the parents, and by means of drugs. Vesani are treated with what he calls specific drugs, with sedativa and with remedies which strengthen the spiritus vitae.

In the case of chorea lasciva, due to excessive rage, the patient was advised to let out all his oaths on a waxen image and subsequently to burn this. If chorea lasciva is due to sexual phantasies, Paracelsus recommends confinement in a dark cell, fasting, " a good stick " and ducking in cold water. These measures can, of course, be regarded as a form of psychotherapy, although Paracelsus explained their effects solely on a physical basis. For chorea originating in the laughing veins, he recommends aurum potabile, ointments, etc. For suffocatio, he prescribes antihelminthics, laxatives, fumigation, ointments and other drugs.

From a study of this work one gains the impression that Paracelsus was a chemical somaticist with occasional psychological and clinical insights (like that of the sexual rather than uterine nature of hysterical seizures). He describes the body as if it were a kind of alchemist's kitchen, in which caustic fumes rise up to cause mental illnesses. This is in no way surprising, since Paracelsus's main contribution to

C

medicine was the introduction of chemical concepts. Neither is it surprising to find that his treatment is not psycho-therapeutic but primarily chemical. The astrological elements of his book are quite concordant with the fashion of his time, in which astrology was regarded as a serious science by the majority of scholars. Despite the occasional appearances of magical elements in it, the book is essentially naturalistic, and Paracelsus' new classification of mental diseases is probably no worse than those of his predecessors. His therapeutic optimism is great and at times comes very near to quackery.

If this were all we knew about the psychiatry of Paracelsus, it would be relatively simple to see it in perspective and to evaluate it as a whole. Unfortunately, however, there is another book by Paracelsus about mental illnesses, called " *The Invisible Diseases* " and written in 1531. In this book chemistry and clinical symptoms are suddenly forgotten; unless we choose to interpret as such his remarks about the influence of the imagination of pregnant women on the formation of the foetus, or his statement that those who kill themselves in despair are inspired by the devil. We now learn that St. Vitus dance, St. Anthony's fire and other such diseases are due to " faith." This book is the work of a mystical philosopher and can be so variously interpreted that every idea entering a physician's head, then, now, or in the future, can be read into it, or picked out from it, without anyone ever being sure what the author really meant.

Furthermore, we find in Paracelsus's " *De Generatione Stultorum* " the first mention of the relationship between goitre and cretinism, and a truly moving appeal for the understanding and humane treatment of " fools." At the same time, however, we find in his " *De Lunaticis* " (Strebel Edition, Vol. 2, page 127-129) the statements that madness can be avoided by means of confession, and that the afflicted should be burned to prevent their becoming tools of the devil. We also find a complete treatise on those possessed by the devil who are not amenable to medical treatment but can only be cured through the power of Christ, by prayer and by fasting. Paracelsus also wrote a book about witches, in which he tells us that they are responsible for thunder storms, that they can produce disease by shooting foreign bodies under the skin (if Australian medicine men were literate, one of them might have written this chapter), and that they are responsible for causing congenital malformations. We also learn that a witch is born as such and that she can be recognised by infallible signs; such as a curved nose, abstinence from sexual intercourse, particularly in the state of widowhood, or by an inclination for intercourse on Saturdays, Fridays and Thursdays.

Paracelsus ends with an appeal in favour of " saving " rather than burning the witches. With these humane and laudable sentiments one can only agree; although they are neither particularly medical nor psychiatric. One can, of course, as has in fact often been done, regard these unbelievable contradictions in Paracelsus's work as signs of his greatness and depth of understanding. It seems to me, however, that there are simpler and more obvious explanations; for example, that he was completely muddled and illogical.

As a campaigner against ancient dogmas, and an unprejudiced observer and chemist, he undoubtedly stood at the cradle of modern medicine and psychiatry. But as a mediaeval mystic and immensely self-contradictory confabulator, he was often forced to support opposing factions; and thus he caused a great deal of confusion.

CHAPTER IV

SEVENTEENTH CENTURY PSYCHIATRY

It was yet another Swiss; Felix Plater (1536-1614), who came forward at the beginning of the seventeenth century and attempted to investigate mental disorders in a new way, more reminiscent of the Greek model. At the very beginning of his " Medical Practice " he devotes several chapters (150 pages in all) to this subject, and his companion volume of clinical observations contains accounts of many interesting cases of mental illness. Plater seems to have had a very strong personal interest in the insane and he used to allow himself to be secluded with his patients. He divides the mental diseases into: (1) imbecilitas; (2) consternatio; which term he uses to describe both the stupor of febrile delirium as well as catatonic states (flexibilitas cerea): his stupor cases include an interesting example of brain tumour discovered at autopsy. Plater was one of the advocates of the use of autopsy to shed light on clinical experience; (3) alienatio; which he divides into dementia; alcoholism, which he also discusses under the headings of imbecilitas and consternatio (one now begins to hear much more about alcoholism following the discovery of distilling processes in the Middle Ages); love and jealousy; melancholia and hypochondriasis; and possession by the devil! Under alienatio he also includes raving mania, St. Vitus dance and phrenitis; (4) defatigatio; whose main manifestation is insomnia, is due to purely supernatural agents (God or the devil) and can, he says, only be treated by corresponding measures. Despite his superstitious prejudices, however, Plater surpassed all his predecessors in the accuracy of his clinical observations. Robert Burton's " *Anatomy of Melancholy* " also appeared for the first time in 1621. This work, which was to become so extremely popular, was in fact simply a collection of classical material, written in the spirit of the times and possessed of certain literary merits. A special form of insanity, dependent upon climate and found particularly among the Swiss, was described in the seventeenth century by J. J. Halder (1678) and J. Hofer (1685) of Basle, under the name of " nostalgia " (home sickness).

On the whole the magnificent developments of psychiatry in the sixteenth century were not followed by steady progress in the next. On the contrary, they faded out. The insane did not yet come under medical care and observation. Although they were again regarded as suffering from mental illness and were no longer punished by death as witches, they were still thought to be incurable, and as such to be outside the field of medicine. This fact seems to me to be the best explanation for the lack of attention paid by seventeenth century physicians to mental diseases. The incurable were, whenever opportunity arose, locked up and chained in prisons, poor-houses, or special institutions. Only in some institutions, like those founded by St. Vincent de Paul (1576-1660) were they treated more humanely. Even in the seventeenth century occasionally the insane were still being diligently burned as witches. It was not until 1680 that a royal edict in France abolished the death penalty for witches. Other countries followed this lead only a century later. Unfortunately we have had to witness yet a further recurrence of mass killing of the mentally sick in the twentieth century; this time in the name of a sort of materialistic religion.

Whilst, therefore, the psychoses were still beyond the reach of medical influence in the seventeenth century, much attention was devoted to another field of mental disturbances, that of the neuroses. Neurotics are, after all, not subject to restrictions of their liberty, and they crowd the doctors' consulting rooms. One might aptly call the psychiatry of the neuroses " out-patient psychiatry." When doctors began to observe these illnesses more closely, the impression was forced upon them that the neuroses were becoming more common. As early as 1600, G. Mercuriali (1530-1606) complained of the increase of hypochondriasis. Thomas Sydenham, the great English clinician (1624-1689), of whom much more will be said later, was of the opinion that half of his non-febrile patients, that is, a sixth of his total practice, were hysterical. In the eighteenth century, George Cheyne (1671-1743), an English clinician, believed that a third of all his patients were neurotic. He actually called his book, published in 1733, the " *English Disease*," and was of the opinion that the English were particularly nervous! With J. G. Zimmermann (1763), already half of the patients were hypochondriacs. Finally, Thomas Trotter (1761-1832), in the early nineteenth century declared that two-thirds of all his patients were neurotic. Trotter had also written a book on alcoholism, a subject which was now receiving more and more attention. From Sydenham onwards the conviction grew in strength that the various symptoms and " diseases " designated as hysterical, hypochondriacal and, later, nervous, covered up some hidden malady but that this was not, as had previously been thought, primarily a disease of the uterus. We thus find a remarkable similarity in the books of Sydenham, Cheyne, Pomme, Trotter, Whytt; and in those of Brachet, Dubois and Louyer-Villermay, up to George Miller Beard's work on neurasthenia, (1880). All attempted to collect the numerous symptoms and to find a common cause for them corresponding to the respective trends of their period.

It seems desirable to present a short abstract of Sydenham's[1] famous notes on hysteria (1680 letter to Dr. Cole); the first, and by no means the worst, of the writings on the neuroses which succeeded one another without interruption until the late nineteenth century. Sydenham regarded hysteria as a most widespread and puzzling disease whose treatment presented the utmost difficulty. According to him, it occurred mainly in women and spared only those women who lead a hard life. Men could also be afflicted and, in particular, those addicted to a sedentary life. In the case of men, the illness was usually called hypochondriasis but it was, in fact, the same as hysteria. The main feature of hysteria was the variety of forms which it could take. Diagnostic errors were, therefore, easily made. It could simulate apoplexy if it occurred after labour or after great excitement. It could take the form of epilepsy, headache, palpitations, cough, " passio iliaca " (chronic appendicitis); of renal colic, diarrhoea, of pain and swelling of muscle; of toothache, backache; of cold in the presence of a normal pulse (the pulse, according to him, remained normal even in cases of hysterical colic or vomiting), and of a feeling of annihilation in the chest. Sydenham (and many of his followers) laid great stress on the production of large amounts of clear urine as a symptom of hysteria. He described hysterics as often being depressed, often, however, boisterous and in general very labile. They always retained their reason. The forms which hysteria could take were so manifold that he considered it impossible to list them all.

Hysteria could be precipitated by excitement; also by prolonged

---

[1] Thomas Sydenham, born 1624 at Wynfort Eagle, Dorsetshire, England, of a Puritan family: father and brother, like himself, were officers in Cromwell's army. 1642, began his studies at Oxford University, but joined the army and returned 1647; 1650 again joined the army; 1656 married and started practising in London; 1659-1661 in Montpellier: influenced by Barbeyrac. Only in 1663 was he made licentiate of the Royal College of Physicians (aged 39). Escaped from the plague in 1665 and wrote his first book on fever, which he dedicated to Robert Boyle and which had an introductory poem by his friend, John Locke. Died of gout in 1689.

fasting or severe blood-letting or purgation. It was due to " ataxia " or " spasmus " of the " spiritus animales," to which Galen and Paracelsus had introduced us. It is interesting to see how Sydenham attempted, in the language of his day, to explain that the illness seemed to him neither purely physical nor purely psychological. Whilst according to Hippocratic tradition he attributed other diseases to the humores, he made an exception in the case of hysteria and called this a disease of the spiritus animales. Women, he said, were more often affected because they were weaker and because their " spiritus " was more delicate. Among Sydenham's many interesting case histories is a most impressive one of a nobleman who suffered from hysterical attacks of weeping.

Sydenham's treatment was simple: He used phlebotomy and purging less often than usual and relied above all on iron preparations, and also on milk diets and on horse-riding which the old cavalry officer held in very high regard. He attempted to suppress attacks by the use of the old, evil-smelling drugs which Aretaeus had already recommended, although for different reasons. He prescribed opium for pain, although he was aware of the risk of addiction.

Another reason for the increasing study of the neuroses in the seventeenth century was the first appearance of neurology on the scene. The great English neuro-anatomist, physiologist and clinician, Thomas Willis (1621-1675), was the first to describe diseases of the nervous system such as myasthenia gravis and dementia paralytica. It is quite wrong that today he should be remembered only by his circle of Willis. His psychiatric methods of treatment, however, were almost brutal. Nevertheless he was one of the first to express the important opinion that hysteria is not a disease of the uterus but of the brain. The same idea had already been voiced by Charles le Pois (1563-1633) in 1618, but with little success; since the view that hysteria is a uterine disease was held by most people until far into the nineteenth century.

It must also be mentioned that blood transfusion, one of the widely practised treatment methods of today, was introduced in the seventeenth century, more or less as a psychiatric treatment method. The Parisian Professor Jean Denis, transferred appreciable amounts of arterial blood from lambs to the veins of mental patients, at first with some success (? due to the effect of shock). Subsequent fatalities led to the prohibition of this procedure. It lay dormant until the surgeons revived it in the nineteenth century, and was not successfully applied until Landsteiner's discovery in the twentieth century of blood groups made its wider use possible.

CHAPTER V

EIGHTEENTH CENTURY PSYCHIATRY

IN the eighteenth century psychiatry at last reached the status of an independent science. Psychiatric achievements surpassed earlier efforts, at first in quantity and later also in quality. This was not primarily due solely to developments in medicine, but to the philosophy of enlightenment which pervaded the whole century. With the spread of enlightenment, belief in possession by evil spirits became just one more manifestation of the detested enemy " superstition " and (with the exception of a few setbacks among the German Romantics of the first half of the nineteenth century), it was now destroyed once and for all. Since the concept of the immortal soul was of no importance in this philosophical system, mental disorders could be viewed as disorders of the mortal brain or thinking apparatus and as such could now at last be studied on a scientific basis. At the same time it became possible to give up a purely somatic viewpoint and to introduce psychology deliberately into psychiatry. Cartesian philosophy, no doubt, played a part in this development.

The growth and development of psychiatry in the eighteenth century was greatly influenced by the deeply philanthropic interests of the philosophers of enlightenment. As reason was their highest good, how they sympathised with those who had lost reason! Their optimism was boundless; as was their belief in attaining human perfection. Thus they overcame the fatalist belief in the incurability of insanity; thus they founded numerous institutions for the mentally sick, and improved the regime within these institutions until the day when, through the great symbolic gesture of taking off the chains of the " mad men," these were definitely reinstated as human beings.

This decisive advance occurred at the end of the century when Abraham Joly in Geneva (1787); Pinel in the Paris Bicêtre (1793); William Tuke, the Quaker, of York (1796); Vincenzo Chiarugi (1759-1820) after 1788 in Tuscany, and John Gottfried Langermann (1768-1852) in 1805 in Bayreuth, struck off the chains from the insane. The prolonged and intensive preoccupation with psychiatry which went

30

on during the whole of the eighteenth century had, of course, prepared the way and provided a basis for this event. As psychiatry was now mainly practised in asylums (which were still outside the universities), the centre of interest shifted once more from the neuroses to the psychoses.

The movement of enlightenment also enabled psychiatrists to demand the right to be heard in the courts. Another result was the new and strong interest taken in the prophylaxis of mental disease. This particular interest was shown by the movement of enlightenment in all fields of medicine and, therefore, also in psychiatry. Enlightenment is, after all, the mother of the social sciences and their application to medicine. The term " sciences sociales " appears for the first time in the *Encyclopédie* of Diderot and d'Alembert and it is not surprising therefore, that in the eighteenth century, for the first time, we come across sociological theories about the causation of mental illness.

The decisive turning point was, no doubt, due to the influence of George Ernst Stahl[1] (1660-1734), the clinician and chemist of Halle. His basic and influential theory of diseases was that of " animism," and it arose as a reaction to iatrophysics and iatrochemistry which predominated at the time. According to Stahl, the chemical and physical reactions of the body are kept going only by means of the soul (anima). Disease, according to him, was a fight between the anima and harmful influences. This view dealt a blow at the old somaticism which had governed psychiatric thinking from Hippocrates to Stahl. Even where somaticism survived, it was in a richer, more complex form. Stahl himself wrote little in any detail about insanity. His basic division of mental illnesses, however, into " sympathetic " (that is, due to disease of organs) and " pathetic " (that is, functional with no organic basis) was widely accepted and was crucial for the whole subsequent development of psychiatry. It is probably also due to Stahl that in the eighteenth century so many men, such as Ch. G. Ludwig (1758), Zueckert (1764), Harper (1789), Fischer (1790), and Langermann (1797), suddenly came forward with theories about the psychogenic causation of mental disease. It is also no coincidence that most of them were German, since it was in Germany that philosophical

---

[1] George Ernst Stahl, born 1660 at Ansbach. After 1694, Professor at the newly-founded university of Halle, together with his friend and later rival, Friedrich Hoffman. 1716, came to Berlin as personal physician to the King of Prussia. Said to have died there in a state of mental confusion in 1734. He was a pietist, invented " animism " in the field of medicine, and the " phlogiston " theory in chemistry, not contested until the time of Lavoisier. Exerted a strong influence on the vitalists of the school of Montpellier.

idealism triumphed in the eighteenth century. The fact that a large part of the so-called psychogenic causes later proved to be false and were found to be symptoms rather than causes of mental illnesses, is here of only secondary importance.

Not only was somaticism accompanied by psychologism in the eighteenth century, it was itself completely changed. Until then somaticists had largely been humoralists, followers of Hippocrates and Galen. But now the basic theories about disease became increasingly more " solidistic," and these conceptions were, of course, shared by psychiatrists. The trends towards solidism and localism were strengthened enormously by the work of the pathological anatomists, above all by that of Morgagni (1761), who performed autopsies on numerous mentally ill patients. This new solidism of the eighteenth century was based especially on the study of the nervous system, about which many important physiological discoveries were now being made. Here, as so often in the history of medicine, new discoveries led to the overemphasis of isolated phenomena and to the development of generalizations derived from these, which were not justified by the facts. The experimental discoveries of Albrecht von Haller (1752) on the sensitivity of the nervous system and on the irritability of muscles (contractibility) were at once converted by Cullen of Edinburgh (1769) into a general explanation of disease as due to nervous disorders. Cullen coined the term " neurosis " and recommended the use of the straight jacket invented by McBride. Robert Whytt's first experiments (1751) with reflexes, which he still called " sympathy," and the experiments by Galvani and Volta (both 1792) with " animal " electricity had similar results. This belated discovery of the nervous system was responsible for the fact that the illnesses which we now call neuroses, and which had until then been thought of as due to " vapours " or to " decay of the humours," were now attributed to the nervous system. Only since the eighteenth century has it been possible to suffer from " nerves."

The eighteenth century also saw the beginning of studies on cerebral localisation (Pourfour du Petit, Lorry, Gall) which were to be of such crucial importance for psychiatry. A product of the late eighteenth century was the medical philosopher, Pierre Cabanis (1757-1802);[2] the

---

[2] Pierre Jean Georges Cabanis, born 1757. At first a writer, 1783 qualified as doctor of medicine in Paris. A friend of Turgot, Madame Helvetius, Holbach, Franklin, Jefferson, Condillac, Diderot, d'Alembert, Condorcet. Together with Destutt de Tracy, leader of the " ideologues " (sensualist philosophers). Concerned with educational reform. Physician of Mirabeau. 1794, professor of

theorist who combined the psychological and somatic points of view, and who exerted a very great influence on medicine, psychiatry, education, politics and even literature of the subsequent decades; despite the fact that today his writings seem full of platitudes. Cabanis belonged to the school of ideologists and became a friend and protector of Pinel. He was one of the later philosophers of enlightenment, and a sensualist. In his famous " *Traité du Physique et du Moral de l'Homme* " (1799), he was primarily concerned to explain " moral," that is, psychological phenomena on a physiological basis. He also demonstrated, however, that moral impressions can have physiologic-pathological results. Thus at last a rational explanation was provided for the psychogenic production of disease, in which the so-called " passions " were held in those days to play a specially important rôle. For the first time also a theoretical explanation was provided for " moral " treatment, that is for psychotherapy. Psychotherapy had after all been theoretically impossible, both on the basis of the older somaticism and on the basis of the old beliefs about the soul. From the middle of the eighteenth century we find an increasing number of books appearing which recommend psychotherapy not only for mental illnesses but also for ordinary physical complaints. We mention here only the works of Bolten (1751), Scheidemantel (1787), Tissot (1782), Falconer (1789), Haslam (1798), and Reil (1803). This was a progressive move despite the fact that one can hardly support the methods of healing by means of fear which were advocated by many writers. It was not until Pinel that fear was banished from the arsenal of psychotherapy. There was, however, a source of psychotherapy in psychiatry, other than the books of learned doctors. Because of the current state of affairs, treatment of the insane was largely in the hands of the chief warders of the institutions and not in those of the physicians. Among these chief warders were many intelligent and humane individuals who discovered, often before the doctors did, that psychotherapy was more effective than the usual methods of purgation and blood-letting.

The eighteenth century in psychiatry is, unfortunately, not only the century of the development of psychotherapy, but also the century of the active development of physical treatment methods which might be regarded as a sort of shock therapy. The old " treatment " by

---

Hygiene at the new Ecole de Santé. 1796, member of the Institute. 1797, professor of clinical medicine. 1798, member of the Council of 500; aided Napoleon in his coup d'état. Member of the Senate and administrator of Parisian hospitals. Later, together with his friends, bereft of his influence by Napoleon. Died 1808.

ducking was supplemented by the so-called Darwin chair (invented by Charles Darwin's grandfather; the physician Erasmus Darwin, 1731-1802). In this chair the insane were rotated until blood oozed from their mouths, ears and noses; and for years most successful cures were reported as a result of its use. Castration and starvation cures were also employed. Old drugs, such as datura and camphor, were introduced once more, and the newly discovered drug, digitalis, was used in large quantities to treat cases of insanity as well as all other types of disease.

The large number of text books which appeared during this period testify to the magnitude of the psychiatric movement in the eighteenth century. We would mention only the works of Battie (1785, he made an early attempt to teach psychiatry in London); of Arnold (1782, he worked on a new classification); Perfect (1787, he was one of the few writers who reported case histories and who tried out treatment with electricity and calomel); Pargeter (1792); Harper (1789); Faulkner (1789); Haslam (1798, he was apothecary to the famous and notorious Bedlam Hospital in London till he was dismissed in 1816); and of Crichton (1798). Great Britain, which was at that time in the forefront of clinical medicine, also produced most of the psychiatric work. But we must also mention the works of French writers; particularly Lorry (1762), Le Camus (1769) and Dufour (1770). Colombier and Doublet (1785), as well as Daquin (1791), attempted even before Pinel to effect reforms in the treatment of mental diseases. Among the writings in the German language, we must refer to those of Auenbrugger, the inventor of percussion (Vienna, 1776). Auenbrugger reported interesting cases of insanity which he attributed to shrinkage of the penis, as it is still done in the case of " Koro " among the Chinese in Java.[3] Furthermore, mention should be made of the books of Greding (1784), Klockhof (1772), Fischer (1790), Langermann (1797), and Reil (1803), who, incidentally, coined the term psychiatry.[4] The first American book on mental diseases, written by the famous Benjamin Rush[5] (*Medical Inquiry and Observations upon the Diseases of the*

---

[3] Ducret, Jos., *Auenbrugger als Psychiater*, Zürich, 1955.

[4] Johann Christian Reil, born 1759 at Rhaude in Ostfriesland. Graduated in Halle, 1782. After 1787, professor there. 1810, professor of Medicine at the newly founded University of Berlin. 1813, died of battle typhus. Vitalist, later " Naturphilosoph," neuro-anatomist. Campaigned unsuccessfully for the foundation of psychiatric institutes in Berlin and Halle.

[5] Benjamin Rush, born near Philadelphia in 1745. Studied and qualified in 1768 in Edinburgh after the six-year apprenticeship which was at that time customary in America. 1769, professor of Chemistry at the newly founded first North

Mind, Philadelphia, 1812), also belongs to eighteenth century currents of thought. Pinel's " *Traité medico-philosophique sur l'Aliénation Mentale*," which appeared for the first time in 1801, represents on the one hand the climax of the eighteenth century, and on the other, the beginning of a new epoch.

Although one cannot help admiring and welcoming the writings of the eighteenth century psychiatrists for their excellent intentions and their progressive views; one cannot ignore the fact that they follow the vogue of their time in their preoccupation with speculation, theories and classifications at the expense of the study and description of concrete case material. The attempt was made only too often to force mental diseases into one of the " systems " so dear to the hearts of the men of the eighteenth century. We have, therefore, not attempted to review any one of these systems. Again, in line with the basic trends of the eighteenth century, many writers were too much preoccupied with disturbances of reason and of intellect, in which they were particularly interested. In this direction, a complete change was to be brought about by Pinel and his school.

American School of Medicine in Philadelphia and, after 1789, professor of Medicine. Very influential teacher. One of the signatories of the Declaration of Independence. Chief physician of Washington's army, 1778, and, after 1799, director of the Mint. Social reformer who campaigned against the death penalty, slavery, alcoholism, maltreatment of the insane, inflation, etc. Famous in medicine, particularly as opponent to the theory of the contagiosity of yellow fever and as an unremitting advocate of blood-letting and purgation. Died 1813.

CHAPTER VI

PINEL, ESQUIROL AND THE FRENCH SCHOOL

PHILIPPE PINEL was born in 1745, the offspring of a family of doctors, in a small village in the South of France. Although originally destined to take up theology, he changed over to mathematics and later to medicine, which he studied in Toulouse and Montpellier. He matured slowly, and in 1778 he moved to Paris. Even then he did not devote himself primarily to the practice of medicine, but to scientific studies, and he earned his living by giving private lessons and by undertaking translations and editorial work. He became a friend of Cabanis and of Thouret, and a member of the salon of ideologists who met at the house of Madame Helvetius. His interest in mental diseases appears to have begun only in the mid-eighties, that is, when he was forty. The revolution which temporarily brought many of his friends to power, also raised the shy and unpretentious Pinel to high positions: In 1793 he was put in charge of the Bicêtre Asylum and in 1795 of the Salpêtrière, where he accomplished his famous work of liberation. Finally, in 1794, he was made Professor of Hygiene and, later, of Internal Medicine in the newly-founded School of Medicine. Among his contemporaries he was known and admired as a physician rather than as a psychiatrist. His *Nosography*, which appeared in 1798, became the bible of the Paris school for twenty years. For us, the predominant interest lies, of course, in his " *Traité médico-philosophique sur l'Aliénation Mentale* " (at first called " *Traité de la Manie* "), which was first published in 1801. In 1822, Pinel was forced into retirement during the purge of the medical school from liberal elements, and he died in 1826.

His *Traité*, which is basic for the newer psychiatry, starts with a critical review of his predecessors. It is characteristic of Pinel that he immediately stresses the achievements of certain warders in reforming the treatment of the insane, in particular those of his collaborator, Pussin, whom in many ways he regarded as his teacher, and that he also emphasises the achievements of his favourite pupil, Esquirol. Equally characteristic is his own description of his work as being philanthropic. Pinel announces that he does not intend to discuss the various hypotheses about the human understanding, its seat and its nature. His task as a natural scientist is, he says, to observe facts and to bring some order into the chaos of the current treatment methods by means of critical and objective (statistical) investigations.

He turns first to the problem of the causation of mental illnesses. He points out that the patient's emotional life is often disturbed before the onset of the actual attack and he emphasises the importance of psychological factors in the development of insanity. Heredity is, for him, the first cause. The second, is harmful factors in the social environment; such as, for example, educational factors. A faulty education can, he says, lead to a true pseudo-dementia. On the other hand, treatment of the insane is, according to him, only a form of education. The third cause is, for him, an irregular way of life. The fourth is what he calls spasmodic passions (rage, fright), and the fifth, enervating or oppressive passions (grief, hate, fear, remorse). He also mentions the dangers of a change-over from an active to an inactive mode of life (the psychological difficulties of retired people were already well known in the eighteenth century), as well as the conflicts between instincts and religious dogma. A sixth cause he sees in the gay passions, and a seventh in the melancholic constitution. Physical factors are mentioned only as the eighth cause, and among these he includes alcoholism, amenorrhoea, non-bleeding haemorrhoids, fever, the puerperium and head injury.

He next presents a general symptomatology of mental diseases. In mania he describes an increase of body temperature, of physical strength, appetite and sexual desire. He frankly discusses the occurrence of masturbation and homosexuality in asylums. Perception of external objects may be disturbed. Thinking may be completely confused, but in cases of so-called "folie raisonnante", thinking remains clear, although the patients are insane. Both Pinel and Esquirol were much preoccupied with such phenomena: this is proof of their final emancipation from the till then prevalent theory of possession; according to which, of course, the insane could only be regarded as suffering from a global disturbance of the mind. In melancholics, thinking is, according to Pinel, completely concentrated on one object. Memory and association of ideas may be disturbed. Pinel here describes a case of aphasia with agraphia and alexia. Disturbances of judgment are particularly striking in folie raisonnante. Dements and idiots can simulate normal powers of judgment because of their imitative faculties.

The main disturbances of the mentally ill are found in the emotional sphere. Raving is far more characteristic of mania than are false ideas or false judgments. The emotional life undergoes a complete change and apathetic stupor may supervene. The imagination may be disturbed as in hypochondriasis; where patients may believe that they have no heart or that their limbs are made of glass or that they have been changed into wolves. The crucial factor is an alteration of character, and a return to the premorbid character is a precursor of recovery.

Pinel then presents his classification of mental diseases. He mocks Cullen and Erasmus Darwin, who looked upon even simple vices as mental illnesses: " Ce serait convertir en petites maisons (private mental hospitals) nos cités les plus florissantes." His classification, on the whole, conforms to the classical models. He recognises only four forms of mental illness: mania, melancholia, dementia and idiocy. There is no parallel in any of our present diseases for his concept of mania or general delirium, which covers essentially all types of agitated states. These, according to Pinel, have their site in the region of the stomach. Plato's old idea was now brought up to date by Cabanis and Pinel, who found the site of mania in the nervous ganglia of the abdominal cavity. In mania, according to Pinel, one sees bizarre, abnormally jolly and also sad behaviour. The course of mania, like that of any acute illness, is self limiting and recovery is often possible; since it is a " purely nervous " disorder not accompanied by organic changes. Mania can also consist of disturbances of the emotional life alone without delirium.

Pinel suggests " exclusive delirium " as an alternative name for melancholia. He rejects too wide an extension of this concept and reserves the term " melancholia " for cases in which the mind is concentrated on a single idea, which may be either sad or grandiose. Melancholics may be mute for years. Melancholia may also degenerate into mania. It often leads to suicide and to the refusal of food, and is characterised by the presence of obsessional ideas and illusions.

Dementia or cessation of thought processes is, above all, the result of exhaustion due to sexual excesses. Thinking becomes quite incoherent, and this distinguishes dementia from mania. In the latter, ideas are false but coherent, whereas in the former they are completely isolated from one another.

In idiocy all intellectual faculties are absent. Cases of idiocy are very common and are often accompanied by alterations in the shape of the skull. They are usually treated too actively. In connection with

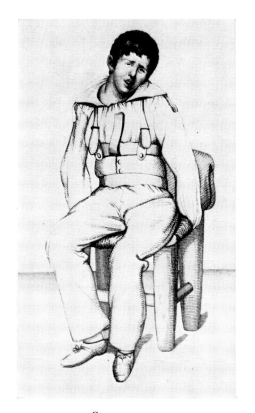

STRAIT-JACKET
(from Esquirol's book)

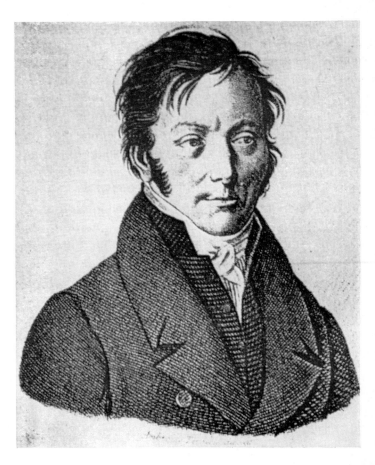

ESQUIROL

idiocy, Pinel makes an excursion into the fields of cretinism and the legal problems of psychiatry.

If we attempt to group the disease pictures recognised today, according to the old classification, we find that " mania " includes cases of schizophrenia as well as hypomania. " Melancholia " includes genuine depressions and also depressed schizophrenics and cases of paranoia, neurosis and general paresis. " Dementia " includes cases of general paresis and late schizophrenics, and " monomania " includes cases of general paresis, paranoia, schizophrenia and neurosis. The old categories are, in fact, not founded on real disease pictures, but on symptomatic states.

Pinel was very much concerned with the principles according to which mental hospitals should be organised and administered. In his hands the hospital becomes the main therapeutic agent. A resolute policy is called for, but at the same time the general attitude should be liberal and such as to inspire confidence. The institutions must, above all, be large enough to allow of segregation of the different categories of patients. He describes the Salpêtrière, with its separate departments for idiots and for thieves; for incurable agitated patients; for curable agitated patients; for quiet patients, dements, senile dements and for convalescents (with workshops). In addition there is a hospital for mentally ill patients who also suffer from other diseases.

He naturally rejects completely the use of chains as a method of correction; having himself abolished them in the Bicêtre and the Salpêtrière. He does resort to the use of the strait-jacket, but warns against using this for too long a period. Both the strait-jacket and the douche may, according to him, be ordered only by the physician. Continuity, the maintenance of a constant routine, and the study of the patient's personality are essential. He regards the division of administrative powers between the medical and administrative heads as one of the major difficulties of hospital organisation; one that has led to an almost grotesque state of affairs in most institutions. Recovered patients, he says, often make good nurses. Food must be distributed with strict fairness. In times of famine the death rate in mental hospitals rises steeply. Physical exercise or mechanical work should, as in Saragossa and Amsterdam, form the basic programme of every mental hospital. Work is of particular importance for idiots. That is why members of the nobility, who reject such activities, are especially difficult to cure. Psychotherapeutic measures must be based on the authority and expert knowledge of the physician, who may sometimes be forced to resort to guile. Religious activities should be carefully restricted, because they sometimes provoke dangerous states of ecstasy. Both Pinel and Esquirol were deeply convinced of the absolute necessity for an early separation of the patient from his family; since the family cannot look after him properly and only produces unnecessary strain. Connections with the outside world in general should be strictly limited. Both in France and in England experience, he says, has shown that too early a resumption of contact with the outside world can lead to dangerous relapses. Some seditious and incorrigible thieves should be nursed apart from the rest of the patients.

The treatment of melancholics demands great skill. Among the case histories presented to illustrate this, one finds, incidentally, cases which we would today classify as paranoia or obsessional neurosis. In cases of food refusal, Pinel introduced tube feeding with great success. He warns against suicide as an ever-present danger, and remarks that it is usually necessary to supervise the hospital staff as carefully as the patients.

Pinel then goes on to review the older and the newer methods used in the treatment of insanity. He rejects beating, which had been liberally used since the time of Celsus, as being ineffective both as a treatment method and also as an educative measure. Neither does he think much of phlebotomy. He refers to sudden ducking, still recommended by Boerhaave, as: " A medical delirium which is more malignant than the delirium of patients." On the other hand, he is a firm believer in the efficacy of baths and also makes moderate use of the douche. In this connection he reports interesting experiments with the douche which Esquirol performed on himself.

It is important to isolate excited patients in the early stages of mania. One must avoid confusing mania with febrile delirium. Fetters should be applied only to the most agitated patients, and then not for long. Patients must be well fed and must have much outdoor exercise. Baths and mild laxatives are helpful. One should always use drugs very sparingly. Melancholia, according to Pinel, is even more difficult to treat than mania; which has a sort of natural course and, therefore, according to Hippocratic theory, a tendency to spontaneous recovery. He stresses the benefits of moral measures of treatment, especially work therapy. Possession and exorcism he regards as nonsense. Pinel prefers more harmless purgatives to the traditional hellebore. He also uses sedatives such as camphor and opium. Mania can sometimes end during a crisis; such as results, for example, from a parotid abscess or a general febrile illness. It is extremely difficult to decide when a case is cured, and the greatest circumspection is indicated at the time of discharge of convalescent patients.

Pinel then presents the results of his statistical investigations, which he considers to be of great importance. Mania he finds primarily between puberty and the age of 45; in women it may begin even earlier. Melancholia is mainly found between the ages of 20 and 40. Of particular importance in melancholia are moral, that is psychological, causes; such as fright, disappointment in love, loss of property, domestic difficulties and exaggerated piety. Among the physical causes, the most obvious ones are constitutional factors, amenorrhoea and the puerperium. He obtains 51% of cures in cases of mania, 62% in melancholia, 19% in dementia, and none at all in cases of idiocy. The average length of treatment is 5½ months in cases of mania, 6½ months in cases of melancholia. He has had 71 relapses among 444 patients. Since most of his incurables received unfavourable treatment elsewhere before coming to him, his results would probably have been even better had they come to him direct. In this connection he makes the interesting observation that if insanity is complicated by paralysis, recovery never occurs.

In incurable cases he thinks that one would probably find organic damage, although the results of morbid anatomical investigations have so far been contradictory. It has often been claimed that abnormalities are found in the abdomen. Skull measurements yield significant results only in cases of idiocy. Moral causes are especially important at certain periods of life or in certain occupations (monks, artists). Physicians and mathematicians rarely become insane. Failure to recover may be due to the onset of other diseases, and here hysteria, epilepsy and hypochondriasis are particularly dangerous. The impossibility of organising work therapy in certain institutions has very unfortunate repercussions. The most difficult patients to treat are the malicious, the wealthy and those accustomed to wield power. Treatment is facilitated to the extent that it can be based on moral values. But progress in ethics has not been as rapid during the eighteenth century as progress in the natural sciences. Educational reform in this direction is most urgent. He hopes that his book will be a contribution to this field in that it demonstrates the tragic results of the neglect of moral values.

In summary, we can say that the most characteristic features of Pinel's psychiatric attitude, which, although rooted in the eighteenth century, marks the beginning of a new epoch, are the following: his indifference to theories and classifications; his strong emphasis on the observation of clinical findings and on statistics; his " Hippocratism," that is, his expectant attitude as an observer; his ethics; his preference for psychogenic aetiological explanations; his fascination by "folie raisonnante," that is, mania without intellectual disturbances; and his " philanthropie " as manifested by his activities as a reformer and humanitarian, his generosity and benevolence and his belief in the possibility of curing mental diseases.   Pinel's strength lay, without doubt, in his gifts as a helper and therapist. He saw himself primarily as a clinician, and from the point of view of formal dogmatism, he was an " eclectic." So were most of the significant psychiatrists after him and this attitude still seems, perhaps because of the youthfulness of psychiatry, to be the most fruitful one; just as it was in the case of internal medicine in a similarly early phase at the time of Boerhaave.

As a physician Pinel had many eminent pupils (Bichat, Broussais, Landré-Beauvais, Schwilguè, etc.).   As a psychiatrist he had only two: Guillaume Ferrus (1784-1861), who earned renown in the field of work therapy and mental hospital reform, and Esquirol.   Jean-Etienne-Dominique Esquirol (1772-1840) came from the same district of France as did Pinel and, like him, he was the son of a doctor, destined to take up theology.   He, also, studied at Toulouse and Montpellier and he, also, entered psychiatry relatively late in life. In 1799 he came to Paris and joined Pinel.   In 1811 he became his colleague on the staff of the Salpétrière.   One can describe Esquirol's basic attitudes in exactly the same terms as those we have just used for Pinel. In spite of this, however, the unique and surprising fact remains that Esquirol was by no means merely a paler edition of his teacher; on the contrary, he was able to achieve even more in the same fields than his master, who was always ready to acknowledge this without a trace of envy. In addition, Esquirol was a gifted teacher. He held the first series of lectures in psychiatry in 1817. He trained many outstanding French and foreign students[1] and was responsible for the pre-eminence of the French School of Psychiatry in the first half of the nineteenth century. His achievements in the field of public health[2] were also quite remark-

---

[1] Lists of the French pupils of Esquirol in *Pariset, E., Eloges*, Vol. 2, p. 476, 482.

[2] See Ackerknecht, E. H., *Hygiene in France* 1815-1848, *Bull. Hist. Med.* 22: 117-55, 1948.

able. In contrast to Laennec, he was popular among his liberal students and colleagues, despite his Royalist views. He had a great love for his profession and for his patients and, like many of his predecessors and many of his successors, he still lived together with his patients. He was, however, greatly hurt by the fact that these, when cured, often behaved in public as if they did not know him. Louis, Leuret, Moreau, Calmeil, Baillarger, and his nephew, Mitivié, gathered around his deathbed, and his last words were: " Live in peace."

Esquirol was a better statistician than Pinel and his clinical observations and descriptions were clearer, more detailed and more exact. Progessive paresis, as well as circular insanity and Jacksonian epilepsy, can be recognised among his descriptions. He also was an " eclectic " and his remark: " Il ne faut jamais être absolu dans la pratique," is epigrammatic. Moreover, he was the more imaginative psychotherapist. He was extraordinarily unbiased and would try out anything that promised some sort of success, even if he distrusted it. This applied to mesmerism, Gall's phrenology, treatment with music, and morbid anatomy. He was, however, not at all enthusiastic about the famous and, at that time, so controversial colony for the insane at Gheel in Belgium, which had sprung up in the former place of pilgrimage. He was free from all prejudices, such as, for example, the still accepted climatism of Hippocrates, or the enlightened anti-clericalism of Pinel. Nor did he succumb to new myths, such as, for instance, that of the " worthy " poor. He freed himself from Pinel's theory of the gastro-intestinal localisation of mania and adopted Gall's theory of cerebral localization. The interpretation of mental illnesses in terms of diseases of the brain is, without doubt, attributable mainly to F. J. Gall, who, despite his " phrenology," made numerous and valuable contributions to the anatomy, physiology and pathology of the brain.[3] Esquirol had a deeper understanding of the " moral " causes of insanity and he recognised that some of the so-called causes, e.g., abuse of alcohol, and masturbation, were often merely early symptoms. He saw much more clearly the roles that social upheavals and the isolation of modern man play in the genesis of mental illnesses. His account is here reminiscent of Stendhal. It is not a coincidence that one of the French terms for mental disease is " aliénation," that is, estrangement. In the course of such diseases, human relationships are disrupted and may even be changed into their opposites. On the other hand, he pointed out how

---

[3] See Ackerknecht, E. H., and Vallois, H. V., *François Joseph Gall et sa collection,* Paris, 1955.

much the mental patient and the normal person have in common, particularly when the latter's attention is distracted. The mental patient loses the capacity for concentration. Esquirol differentiated between hallucinations and illusions. His work on the subject of hallucinations was continued by Alexandre Brierre de Boismont (1798-1881), who did much work with criminals. Esquirol developed Pinel's ideas about " folie raisonnante " in his teaching about the monomanias or partial insanities, which was, however, rejected by many of his pupils, e.g., J. P. Falret, Trélat, Foville. Another name he gave to melancholia was lypemania, and he followed Pinel in thinking that the content of delirium in these cases consists only of a single object.

Esquirol also discussed at length, and with the use of statistics, the still unsettled problem of whether mental diseases are increasing in our culture. Esquirol believed that any increase was more apparent than real. An answer to this problem would, of course, also answer the question as to whether civilisation produces more mental ill-health than other forms of culture. In the light of this discussion it becomes at once apparent why medical men of different nationalities have from time to time (in England in the eighteenth, in America in the nineteenth century) pointed almost with pride to their wealth of neurotics. If civilisation produces mental diseases, then the country with the largest number of patients must be the most civilised.

Esquirol the reformer was no less successful than Esquirol the research worker. The French legal code of 1838, relating to administration of mental health, was designed by him and is the first comprehensive legislation in this field (a partial law had existed in England since 1828). It served as a model for similar legislation in Switzerland (1838), England (1842), and Norway (1848). His private sanatorium in Ivry and his institution at Charenton, which were built according to his own plans and which he administered from 1826, were model institutions. Charenton (at present under the direction of Professor Baruk, who lovingly guards Esquirol's beautiful library) is, to this day, a remarkable place. The asylums in Saint-Yon, Le Mans, Montpellier and Marseilles were also built according to his plans. In this connection, attention should be drawn to the fact that special institutions were at last being created for the care of feeble-minded and idiots. J. E. Belhomme (1824) was the first to found such an institution, and he was followed by Ferrus (1828); Felix Voisin (1834); and Eduard Seguin (1839), whose work in America after 1848 developed in a most fruitful way. A special role was played between 1826 and 1893 by the private institution in Paris run by Dr. Esprit Blanche[4] and his son, Emile. Here many mentally ill " gens du monde," and especially artists, from Nerval to Maupassant found a place of asylum. Esquirol's influence continued to be felt until the eighties of the last century because of his pupils; J. J. Moreau de Tours (1844-1884), about whom more will be said in connection with the degeneration theory; and J. Baillarger (1809-1890), to whom we owe, among other things, the recognition in 1854 of circular insanity as a definite disease picture and who, in 1850, described the pupillary changes in general paresis. Baillarger and Moreau, together with Cérise and Brierre, were also responsible for establishing the important " Annales médico-psychologiques " in 1843.

Of the other pupils of Esquirol, only the most important can be mentioned. Etienne Jean Georget (1795-1828), his favourite student, the friend of the painter, Guericault, died young. His main work dealt with legal psychiatry and the cerebral localization of all mental diseases, including hysteria. The preface to his " Physiologie du système nerveux " sounds like a preliminary study to Claude Bernard's " Intro-duction à la Médecine Expérimentale." François Leuret (1797-1851) became the advocate of a generally rather foolish type of " moral " treatment, and thus took a step backwards to the time before Pinel. His clear-sighted psychological observations, however, were still quoted by Freud and Janet. Jean-Pierre Falret (1794-1870), who must not be confused with his son, Jules (1824-1902), began his work with studies on suicide; a subject which has always held a particular fasci-nation for French sociologists and psychiatrists. He began as a somaticist, but his attitudes became more and more those of a psycho-logist. Had it not been foreign to his nature, he might have defended his rightful claim to the two great French discoveries of dementia paralytica and circular insanity. He began an important social inno-vation; insurance for discharged patients (1843). Together with his friend, Felix Voisin (1794-1872), not to be confused with the latter's nephew, Auguste Voisin (1829-1898), he founded the famous private institution in Vanves. Voisin, who was much influenced by Gall, devoted himself above all to the study and training of the feeble-minded. Achille Foville (1799-1878) is renowned mainly for his neuro-anatomical studies. Louis Florentin Calmeil (1798-1895), another pupil of Esquirol,

---

[4] Le Breton, J., La Maison de Santé du Docteur Blanche, Paris Th. 1937.

was one of the first to recognise dementia paralytica as a separate disease (1826) and is the author of a classic history of mass psychoses. Antoine Laurent Bayle (1799-1858) was a nephew of the clinician Gaspard Laurent Bayle, a protégé of Laennec and a pupil of A. Royer-Collard. In his doctorate thesis of 1822 he had already attributed dementia paralytica to a chronic meningitis and had described its various stages.

Although, as Henri Ey has shown,[5] differences between the psychological and the somatic orientations are noticeable in France, too, they never developed there into a fundamental dichotomy as they did in Germany at that time. Among those with a psychological orientation were Pinel, Fodéré, Esquirol, Lélut, Falret, Baillarger and especially the Belgian, Guislain. Those who thought primarily along somatic lines included Ferrus, Calmeil, Prost, Georget, Bottex, Voisin, Foville and Moreau. The strength of the somatic orientation can be traced as much to the then very powerful influences of Gall and Broussais,[6] as to the contemporaneous successes in the field of morbid anatomy of the nervous system achieved by Rostan, Lallemand, Bouillaud, Andral, Rochoux, Parent-Duchatelet and Martinier and, above all, by Bayle and Calmeil. The materialistic tradition in French philosophy also played its part. Finally the somatic orientation gained the upper hand in France as elsewhere, and assumed the peculiar form of the degeneration theory.

In this same period Great Britain produced only one psychiatrist of note. This was the Quaker, James Cowles Prichard (1785-1848), also known as an anthropologist. He struggled with the same problem of " monomania " as did Pinel and Esquirol and created the category of " moral insanity." The great English contribution to international psychiatry of that time was the introduction of the system of " no restraint." Robert Gardner Hill and Charlesworth had started it at Lincoln in 1829 and John Conolly (1794-1866)[7] led the campaign after 1839 at Hanwell.

[5] Ey, H., *Etudes Psychiatriques*, Vol. 1, p. 34, Paris, 1948.

[6] Ackerknecht, E. H., *Broussais*; *Bull. Hist. Med.* 27: 320-43, 1953.

[7] John Conolly, born 1794 at Market Rasen, Lincolnshire. At first a soldier. Spent some time with his brother, William, a practitioner in Tours, France. Did not begin medical studies until 1817 in Edinburgh. 1821-27, country doctor. 1828, Professor of Practical Medicine at University College, London. 1830-38, Warwick. After 1839, physician to Hanwell, a large mental hospital near London. Prolific writer and one of the founders of the British Medical Association. Died 1866.

CHAPTER VII

THE THEORY OF DEGENERATION

ABOUT the middle of the nineteenth century, the somaticists went through a period of disillusionment. Except in the senile psychoses and in general paralysis, the results obtained from anatomical studies of the brain had not come up to expectation. In contrast to the diseases of heart, lungs, intestines, etc., no objective foundation had been found for the symptoms of mental disease. A new idea was then advanced—the degeneration hypothesis[1]—which seemed to solve the problem of " somaticism ": it held out hopes of establishing unequivocal physical signs of mental illness, more tangible than the variable changes hitherto demonstrated in the brain, and hopes, too, of synthesising all known facts and finally arriving at an aetiological rather than a symptomatic classification of mental disorders. This idea came to the fore almost at the same time as the Darwinian theory, and because it could so readily be brought into line with Darwinism, it gained enormous popularity among psychiatrists, as well as in all classes of the general population. However attractive in its own right, the degeneration hypothesis would never have acquired the significance it did if it had not coincided with the Darwinian theory, then sweeping all before it. From the therapeutic standpoint, degeneration was a pessimistic idea, but the philosophy of the period was predominantly pessimistic; so also was the climate of thought among psychiatrists, working as they did almost entirely in mental hospitals with what seemed to be mostly hopeless cases.

This important concept originated in France. It developed from ideas about heredity and mental illness which were already old and which had been held by Perfect, Burrows, Pinel, Esquirol, Marc, Falret père and Baillarger. Rush, Kirkbride and Woodward had, it is true, greatly restricted the part played by heredity; reflecting no doubt the lack of sympathy which Anglo-Saxons in general have always shown

---

[1] In the preparation of this chapter I have drawn largely from the excellent book, by Georges Genil Perrin: " *Histoire des Origines et de l'évolution de l'idée de dégénérescence en médecine mentale.*" Paris, 1913.

towards " pessimistic " studies such as those on heredity or constitution. Prosper Lucas's work: " *Traité philosophique et physio-
logique de l'hérédité naturelle*" (Paris, 1847), had given great impetus
to genetic research in psychiatry. The theory of degeneration had
already been formulated by J. Moreau de Tours (1804-1884), who since
1850 had been shifting the emphasis in aetiology towards a multiform
hereditary predisposition; which could, for example, account also for
scrofula and rickets and which could be recognised by so-called
stigmata. His experimental work on hashish was of more value and
led him to describe insanity as a " rève éveillé."

The real creator of the degeneration theory was Benedict Augustin
Morel (1809), who was born in Vienna of French parents. Morel and
his friends Claude Bernard, Lasègue and Davaine, were penniless
medical students who had to earn their living by giving private lessons.
Bernard had introduced Morel to Jean Pierre Falret, whose pupil
he became. In addition to these influences, Morel was greatly impressed
by the anthropological studies of Gall, Blainville, Flourens and Serres.
With Buchez and Cérise, he belonged to a small group of medical men
who combined political radicalism with most devout Catholicism and
were the pioneers of social orientation in medicine.

His theory of degeneration reflects all these influences. The hypothesis is at once psychiatric and socio-anthropological. To him,
degeneration is as much a religious as a scientific concept, and in this
he differs as much from the older naturalists, Buffon and Blumenbach,
who used the term to mean variation, as from the newer biologists like
Heusinger, to whom it meant atavism. To Morel, as a pious Christian,
such concepts were foreign. He defines degeneration as follows: " Les
dégénérations sont des déviations maladives du type normal de
l'humanité, héréditairement transmissibles et évoluant progressive-
ment vers la déchéance." (Degenerations are deviations from the normal
human type, which are transmissible by heredity and which deteriorate
progressively towards extinction). Morel worked on this problem
from 1839 onwards, and gave it its final form in the " *Traité des
Dégénérescences Physiques, Intéllectuelles et Morales de l'Espèce
Humaine*," which appeared in 1857. According to him, degeneration
could be caused by: (1) intoxication (malaria, alcohol, opium, soil
conducive to cretinism, epidemics, food poisoning); (2) the social
milieu; (3) pathological temperament; (4) moral sickness; (5) inborn
or acquired damage; (6) heredity. The combined effect of physical
and moral injuries was particularly dangerous (" law of two-fold

fertilisation "). Degeneration was also subject to the "law of pro-
gressivity." The first generation of a degenerate family might be merely
nervous, the second would tend to be neurotic, the third psychotic,
while the fourth consisted of idiots and died out. Because such diseases
and diseased families were becoming more frequent, modern society
was inevitably approaching extinction. By means of a very hazy
concept of "heredity predisposition," Morel was able to attribute the
most diverse illnesses in one generation to the occurrence of quite
different illnesses in the preceding generation: "All hereditary illnesses
are sisters."

The degenerative illness par excellence was insanity, although Morel
admitted the existence of a small number of mental illnesses which
were not degenerative. He claimed to have determined changes in the
head, eye, ear, genitalia and intestines which were infallible stigmata
of degeneration. On the basis of his theory, Morel created a new and,
according to him and his friends, aetiological classification of the insane
into: impulsive eccentrics, "manie raisonnante," instinctive maniacs,
idiots and cretins. Morel not only influenced Griesinger, but also
found devoted followers in Germany in R. von Krafft-Ebing (1840-
1902), best known for his studies of sexual perversions; and H. Schuele,
through whom he influenced German psychiatry for several decades.
These wildly exuberant theories did not prevent Morel from being an
outstanding clinician and diagnostician.

His ideas were taken up in France and after 1870 were developed in
particular by Valentin Magnan (1835-1916). Magnan discarded the
religious side of Morel's concept and interpreted degeneration as
regression in the Darwinian sense. Because of Magnan's immense
prestige, judged by some to equal that of Kraepelin, the idea of degeneration dominated French psychiatry for several decades. Magnan had
first studied degeneration in alcoholics; he also performed useful
animal experiments in alcoholism. The predominant interest of
psychiatrists of this period in alcoholism (see also, e.g., Forel, Bleuler,
Kraepelin) and the degeneration hypothesis are closely related. Magnan
came to the conclusion that all obsessions and compulsive neuroses
and all delusional states were syndromes of degeneration. He also
believed in numerous anatomical, physiological and intellectual
stigmata. At the same time, he put forward an interesting three-level
theory of nervous physiology and pathology (first level, intellect, i.e.
cerebral cortex; second level, sensitivity, i.e. basal ganglia; third level,
spinal) which is extraordinarily reminiscent of the ideas of his con-

temporary, John Hughlings Jackson (1834-1911), the English neurologist. In degeneration, according to Magnan, the equilibrium between the three levels was disturbed.

The heyday of the degeneration hypothesis coincided closely with the vogue for discussing the relationship between genius, insanity and crime. Felix Voisin (" *Des Causes Morales et Physiques des Maladies Mentales*," Paris, 1826, p. 4), a pupil of Gall, had already drawn attention to this relationship: a connection between mental illness and genius had been repeatedly postulated since the days of Aristotle. Moreau de Tours, one of the fathers of the degeneration theory, took up the question again in " *La Psychologie Morbide dans ses Rapports avec la Philosophie de l'Histoire* " (1859). Genius for him was simply a neurosis. Magnan followed his lead. The degeneration theory seemed to provide a simple explanation for this relationship. Both the genius and the madman were degenerates, with the difference that the genius was a " dégénéré supérieur." At this stage, Lombroso (1864) and Max Nordau appeared on the scene and dealt with the same question in their popular books which met with such tremendous acclaim. (For a more recent and unusually thorough study of the problem itself, see W. Lange-Eichbaum: " *Genie, Irrsinn und Ruhm*," Munich, 1956).

People had believed in a criminal physiognomy, too, since Aristotle. Vauvenargues and Cabanis had already identified crime with madness. Gall had regarded a large proportion of criminals as congenital, had found in them certain physical stigmata, and had suggested reforms of the penal code which later became famous in association with the name of Lombroso. Here again the theory of degeneration gave new impetus to consideration of the problem. Morel and Moreau believed that the same hereditary predisposition was present in criminals and in the insane, and in both it was, of course, a matter of degeneration. Only then did the Italian psychiatrist, Cesare Lombroso (1836-1909), take up the question in his " *Uomo delinquente* "; thus becoming the creator of " criminal anthropology." His own contribution consisted solely in his interpreting degeneration on evolutionary lines, as atavism, so that he regarded criminals as a kind of surviving primitive race. Rarely has a psychiatrist achieved such fame on the strength of other men's ideas.

Towards the end of the century the degeneration theory began to lose credit in psychiatric circles. Ziehen and Kraepelin, although still much influenced by it, restricted it greatly. Konrad Rieger (1855-1939) opened the direct offensive against it (1892). The work of Stieda and

Schwalbe showed that many " stigmata " were simply variations with no pathological significance; the comparative studies of Diem and Jenny Koller discredited certain false ideas about heredity which had made even progressive paralysis a degenerative hereditary disease. Experience failed to confirm the concept of progressive degeneration either in families or in nations.

The degeneration theory of " polymorphous " heredity was finally exploded by the new and more accurate knowledge of the actual mechanisms of heredity, which spread rapidly as a result of Mendel's experimental work and its revival at the beginning of the twentieth century. The beautiful dream of a new synthesis was over. The works of Genil-Perrin (1913) and Oswald Bumke (1912) can be regarded as the epitaph of the classical degeneration theory. The pseudo-problem of degeneration gave way to the real, difficult, and still much debated problem of the inheritance of mental illnesses, from which it had originally sprung. Regrettable and unscientific by-products of heredity studies; such as the Nazi law " for the prevention of hereditarily tainted progeny " have disappeared too. The curious concept of degeneration, which had raised so many hopes in psychiatry and met with such unexpected acclaim, still remains alive in the mind of the general public, and also re-emerges from time to time, under various guises, in scientific works.

Darwin's and Herbert Spencer's concept of evolution had not only made the degeneration theory popular, but also stimulated the English neurologist, John Hughlings Jackson, to explain epilepsy on the basis of an evolutionary three-level theory of the central nervous system (lowest level, spinal cord and medulla; second level, basal ganglia; third level, frontal cortex): in epilepsy and mental illness there was cessation of function of an upper level of the central nervous system and continued function of a lower level. Jackson's theory, which was not entirely new, exerted a tremendous influence on neurophysiology, neurology and psychiatry from the turn of the century. It was influential even in such specialties as psychoanalysis and " psychosurgery "; particularly since it seemed to be borne out by the large-scale observations made on post-encephalitic states after 1918. Jackson's theories constituted probably the most successful application to medicine of the concept of evolution.

CHAPTER VIII

GERMAN PSYCHIATRY OF THE FIRST HALF OF THE NINETEENTH CENTURY

WE turn now to German psychiatry, which was to take the international lead in the second half of the nineteenth century. In the early nineteenth century German psychiatry, like German medicine in general, was dominated by the spirit of romanticism. August Hirsch went so far as to consider it to be the best part of German romantic medicine. The Germans had, as nations often seem to do, reacted to the ravages of two defeats; the first an external one, the second internal, with an intensive flight into metaphysics and mysticism. It is no coincidence that so many psychiatrists of this period were poets, nor that at this time Paracelsus's reputation in Germany underwent a radical change. Kurt Sprengel had still discussed him quite soberly. One can hardly say that this new trend in German medicine and psychiatry was a profitable one, particularly if one compares its results with those achieved in France by other means at the same time. It cannot be denied that some fruitful and even some brilliant ideas lie hidden in the morass of romantic concepts, but it requires almost superhuman efforts, of which only few are capable, to disentangle these ideas from the speculative and moralistic verbiage of the period. The temptation has always existed to conceal ignorance beneath a cloak of empty and exotic (or esoteric) words, instead of admitting it with frankness and with humility; but rarely has it been so much indulged as in this era.

The romantic movement in psychiatry found its purest expression in the psychicists; so called because they regarded mental illnesses as diseases primarily of a disembodied soul. They engaged in bitter strife with the somaticists who, for their part, treated mental illnesses as if they were exclusively bodily disorders with more or less important psychological symptoms. It is as well that the romantics were known by the special name " psychicists," because it would certainly be wrong to regard them as psychologists. What they called psychological was largely moralistic, whereas, strangely enough, what the French in this period designated as " moral " was largely psychological.

Many leaders of the romantic movement in medicine, e.g.; Windischmann, Leupoldt or Ringseis, looked upon every illness as the result of sin.[1] The most prominent representative of this movement in psychiatry was J. Heinroth (1773-1843), whose textbook appeared in 1818. He regarded mental disease purely as a disease of the soul and essentially as a " lack of freedom." God had punished the sinner by depriving him of his freedom of will. With such a piece of sophistry, this curious psychiatrist came to the conclusion that the mentally ill are, in fact, responsible for their actions. Logically enough, he rejected hereditary factors as playing a part in mental diseases, because each individual is always provided with a new soul. Despite his occasionally brilliant but soon forgotten aperçus, it would be incorrect to regard him as one of the fathers of psychosomatic medicine, although he did coin the word. His importance lies rather in the fact that he took over developmental ideas along with other romantic speculations and applied them to psychiatry. Some of his formulations are impressive, e.g.; " Wie der Mensch liebt, so lebt er." Heinroth also concerned himself with classification (" the science of form ") and found thirty-six different kinds of mental illness. Apart from the religious, there were the ethical psychicists, such as K. Ideler (1795-1860). Ethical insight and behaviour were for him the ultimate criteria of mental health. Mental disease was brought about by unbridled passions and was the expression of an extreme degree of individuality. A further group of psychicists consisted of the psychologists, such as F. E. Beneke (1798-1854), who worked with such speculative concepts as changes in the boundaries of the soul. Others, such as Haindorf and Kieser, gave themselves up to general romantic speculations about polarity, etc. The regressive element of romantic psychiatry is most clearly illustrated by the fact that Justinus Kerner (1786-1862) and K. K. Eschenmeyer (1768-1852) went so far as to revive the concept of possession and once more to recommend exorcism. Kraepelin explained the romantic movement in psychiatry on the basis of a lack of experience. This may have been true for some of its representatives. It was certainly not true for a great many of them. They were all familiar with the great French collections of empirical material. The fact remains that despite their occasional expressions of approval of knowledge gained from expe-

---

[1] See also Siebenhaar, W. von., *Krankheit als Folge der Sünde*, Hanover, 1950.

rience, this was for them of less importance than their idealistic constructs.

The somaticists, e.g. Friederich Nasse (1778-1851), had a much more down-to-earth approach. Nasse continued indefatigably in his task of founding psychiatric periodicals, which his teacher, Reil, had begun in 1805. Nasse worked especially on the psychological functions of the heart. J. B. Friedreich (1796-1862) worked on the basis of the old theory which has meanwhile once more become fashionable; that psychopathy is based on temperament. Maximilian Jacobi (1775-1858) was interested in all somatic manifestations of mental disease, especially in pulse rate and chemical changes. He had several very gifted pupils, among them F. Bird. His " Observations " appeared in 1830. As Joachim Bodamer rightly pointed out in connection with Nasse and Jacobi, even the somaticists, and later even Griesinger, showed some romantic idealistic traits.[2] Thus they arrived at their somaticism only because they were convinced that the immortal soul could not become diseased. Fundamentally, the somaticist and the psychicist movements were equally speculative[3] and equally unfruitful. It would not be fair to look for the roots of psychicism only in the spirit of the age. It flourished in part because of the sterility of somaticism.

Groos and Blumroeder attempted a speculative mediation between the psychicists and the somaticists. Even in Feuchtersleben's (1806-1849) late attempt at a compromise, one can still clearly distinguish the moralistic and metaphysical elements of romanticism. Apart from this, Feuchtersleben worked largely on the basis of the concept of coenaesthesia (inner sensory impressions) which had been current in France since the time of Cabanis. The concept of coenaesthesia was used to link up purely external influences with spontaneous psychic activity.

German administrative psychiatry flourished during this period. Modern institutions were opened everywhere, e.g.; in 1811 Sonnenstein, in 1825 Siegburg (under the direction of Jakobi), in 1834 Sachsenberg (under the direction of K. Flemming, 1799-1880), in 1834 Winnenthal (Superintendent, A. Zeller, 1804-1872, Griesinger's teacher), in 1836 Halle (under the direction of H. Damerow, 1798-1886, a pupil of

---

[2] Bodamer, J., Zur Phänomenologie der geschichtlichen Geistes in der Psychiatrie; Nervenarzt, 19: 229-310, 1848.

[3] Birnbaum, K., Geschichte der psychiatrischen Wissenschaft. in Bumke, O., Handbook of Mental Diseases; Vol. I, p. 30, Berlin, 1928.

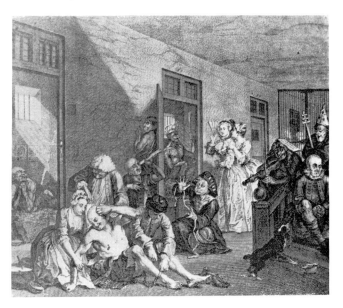

BEDLAM as seen by HOGARTH

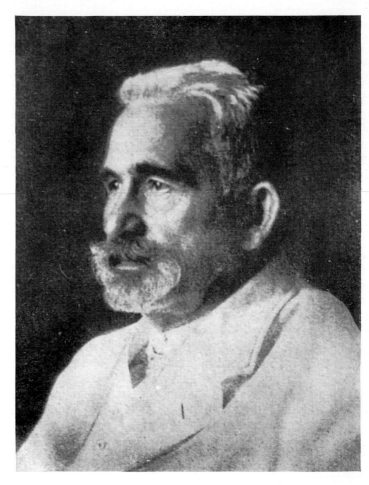

EMIL KRAEPELIN

Esquirol), in 1842 Illenau (Superintendent, Christian Roller, 1802-1878). Guggenmoos, the teacher (1816 in Salzburg), opened the first school for cretins, and J. Guggenbühl (1816-63) built in 1840 on the Abendberg near Interlaken, the first institution for cretins. Thus, the directors of institutions, whose speculations were constantly exposed to the test of reality through their daily contact with the patients among whom they lived, became the leading forces of German psychiatry[4] between 1830 and 1860. Three of the best known of them (Damerow, Roller and Flemming) founded the " *Allgemeine Zeitschrift für Psychiatrie* " in 1844; taking as their model the French " *Annales* " with whose editors they were in close contact. This was the first German psychiatric journal which was to survive. Except for the somaticist, Flemming, their philosophy was an anthropological one based on the unity of mind, body and soul; that is, they formed a transitional generation between the romantics and the mechanists.

Griesinger was responsible for the victory of mechanism. German " institutional psychiatry " was overshadowed by German " university psychiatry," and, as such, attained international fame and significance.[5] This transition also took place in France, but occurred later and was there less conspicuous.

The use of all-too-active treatment methods persisted into the first half of the nineteenth century and included the revolving chair, to which the most varied names were applied. " Nausea " and " pain " therapies were also used, as was the douche. E. Horn (1774-1848), who is regrettably famous for his special sack and his method of forced standing, used to drench his patients at the Charité at Berlin with not less than two hundred pails of water at one sitting.

Wilhelm Griesinger was born in Stuttgart in 1817. During his high school years and his student years at Tübingen he became a close friend of the surgeon, Roser, and the internist, Wunderlich. Together with them he was to found the " *Archiv für physiologische Heilkunde* " in 1842, which became one of the most important agents in the reform of German medicine in the mid-nineteenth century. After studying at Tübingen and Zürich, Griesinger worked for two years with Zeller at Winnenthal. On the basis of his experience there, he published the first edition of his " *Pathologie und Therapie der Psychischen Krank-*

---

[4] Bodamer, J., *Zür Entstehung der Psychiatrie als Wissenschaft im* 19. *Jahrhundert. Fortschr. d. Neurologie-Psychiatrie*, 21: 511-34, 1953.
[5] K. Jaspers is responsible for the concepts of " Institutional Psychiatry " and " University Psychiatry ": see his brilliant historical chapter in his " *Allgemeine Psychopathologie*," Berlin-Heidelberg, 1948, pp. 703-716.

heiten " in 1845.   The last edition to appear in his lifetime was that of
1867.   In 1843 he was made Professor of Internal Medicine at Tübingen, and in 1849 at Kiel.   From 1850 to 1852 he was physician to
the Egyptian Khediv and Director of Medical Services at Cairo.   His
famous book on infectious diseases (1857) is based on his experiences
there.   After again holding the chair of Internal Medicine at Tübingen
and Zürich, he moved to Berlin in 1865, where he became Professor
of Psychiatry and Neurology and where he died at an early age in
1869.

Griesinger begins his " *Pathologie und Therapie der Psychischen
Krankheiten* " (Translation by C. C. Robertson, *New Sydenham Society
Publications*, No. 33, London, 1862) with a plea for the localisation
of mental diseases and their symptoms.   There is no doubt in his
mind that the brain is the seat of mental diseases, although it has
not yet been possible to discover specific brain damage corresponding
to individual mental disorders: " Psychische Krankheiten sind Erkran-
kungen des Gehirns " (" Psychological diseases are diseases of the
brain "), " Das Irresein ist nur ein Symptomenkomplex verschiedener
anomaler Gehirnzustaende" (" Insanity is merely a symptom-complex
of various anomalous states of the brain ").   Unfortunately, he said,
the knowledge of cerebral disorders is still in the stage of the knowledge of respiratory diseases before the time of Laennec.   Of course
not all cerebral diseases manifest themselves as mental diseases.   The
diffuse cerebral disorders are most likely to do so.   Psychiatry must
become an independent discipline and its attitude must be a medical
one and not poetic or moralistic.   Although he recognised psychological
causes for mental diseases, he warned against over-rating them at the
expense of physical causes.

In his " physiopathological preamble " he states that all sensory
impressions are transmitted to the brain, where they are converted into
concepts, general pictures and abstractions.   Concepts in Herbart's
sense can also arise from within the brain.   One may be quite unconscious of such concepts, indeed the larger and more important part of
mental events is unconscious.   Protracted mental impressions or
concepts can evoke complementary phenomena, just as is the case in
prolonged sensory stimulation.   Memory is the reproduction of old
concepts by means of an association of ideas.   The function of reason
depends largely upon that of memory.

Cerebral irritation leads to abnormal concepts and actions. Irritation
of the contents of the abdominal cavity can result in cerebral irritation.

(This is almost pure Broussaisism: Not in vain had Griesinger spent two prolonged periods in Paris). These irritations lead at first to emotional rather than intellectual disturbances.

It is valid to compare psychological pain, a basic phenomenon of mental illnesses, with physical pain. Psychological pain depends upon cerebral irritability. An inflamed nerve is sensitive even to very small stimuli. Psychological pain is a " sensory " phenomenon. The patient invents false concepts (deliria) in order to explain this pain. The " sensory " experiences then result in appropriate motor, i.e. willed, behaviour. The instincts are found at an intermediate level between simple reflex actions and behaviour which results from these complicated sensory-motor relationships. In insanity, instincts are uncontrolled.

Just as Romberg had based his classical text-book of mental diseases (1840) on Bell and Magendie's discoveries (1822) about sensory and motor tracts, so Griesinger based his system of psychiatry, which is essentially a form of reflex theory, upon the same discoveries and upon Marshall Hall's subsequent experimental investigations and findings about reflexes.

In the exposition of his views, Griesinger passes imperceptibly from anatomy to physiology and thence to psychology—his " ego " psychology. He describes different developmental stages of the " ego," which he regards as being made up of a number of different conceptual elements. The ego, according to him, develops into a specific structure. It is, in the healthy state, capable of reflection. A man with a happy nature is one who finds it easy to harmonise the many different traits of his ego (e.g. a religious man or an empiricist), and to play any of the rôles potentially present in his ego. If the ego becomes sick as a result of new sensory impressions, drives and concepts, it reacts at first by resisting these new and pathological ideas with a strong and usually sad emotion. Gradually, however, the ego gives up the struggle, becomes changed and finally destroyed. Once the ego has undergone a structural change, recovery is impossible. Only a strong ego is free; that is, responsible in the legal sense. Griesinger here talks in terms of psychic tonus, of faster and slower contractions. He discusses the two-way relationship between affective and somatic changes. The strongest affects, such as fear and fright, are both somatic and psychological in nature. Emotions, which can precipitate bodily illnesses or can make them worse, can also be caused by them, and herein lies the key to the complex development of what we call mental diseases.

In the insane, certain moods, sensations and decisions arise from within and are not based on external stimuli, as in the normal person. At times, however, such unmotivated states of grief, gaiety and excitement are known to occur also in health. This gives us some understanding of the patient, although several of his experiences are not accessible to the normal person.

After this survey, Griesinger begins his detailed analysis of disturbances of mood, thinking, will, sensations and motor behaviour. Mental disturbances, he says, often begin with states of fear. A happy madness often follows states of depression; the patient becomes irritable, his character alters, he becomes blunted, his relationships with others are changed.

Disturbances of thinking include retardation, and quickened, confused thought; memory often remains unimpaired. If hallucinations occur, these follow the trends of the patient's original concepts; whether he believes he is being persecuted by witches, freemasons or magnetists, depends upon his educational level and his attitudes to life. Following disturbances of emotion, the patient develops deep-rooted and false ideas and his condition becomes stationary. All fixed ideas are ideas of reference and are the expression either of a limitation (which was even at that time translated into the English word " frustration ") or a gratification of the patient's mood and wishes. Many historical ideas which appear to us to be delusions (e.g. a belief in witchcraft) were not the result of mental diseases. Their psychological basis was completely different. Griesinger criticises Esquirol's idea of monomania. He holds that the psychological unity is always destroyed, even if formal examination reveals only a disturbance of part functions.

Disturbances of the will vary from its total absence (stupor) to over-activity and ecstasy. Griesinger again compares this situation with the reflex. He mentions Leubuscher's abulia. Instinctual drives towards motor activity are powerful. The question of legal responsibility (absence of free will) is concerned not so much with automatic, compulsive behaviour, as with states of great excitement or upsetting perceptual disturbances. Griesinger here once more draws a parallel between normal and pathological events in the psychic life and discusses kleptomania as described by Jacobi.

As far as the primary disturbances of perception are concerned, the patient may feel himself to be ill or well. Often he has the feeling that the body he inhabits is not his own. Areas of anaesthesia are frequently found, and not only in hysterics. Hallucinations and illusions are, of course, typical disturbances in the perceptual sphere. Hallucinations are certainly in part organically determined, but can also occur in normal people. He refers here to Pascal, Spinoza, Goethe, Jean Paul, Walter Scott, Johannes Mueller, Andral and many others.

Many states occur in the normal person which are analogous to states of insanity; for example, the dream, febrile deliria and states of intoxication. Both in the dream and in the delirium of mental disease, a person reacts unknowingly to bodily sensations. In both states the person has lost his critical faculties. In the dream, as well as in the delirium of the insane, we can observe the gratification of wishes which in reality had been unfulfilled and repressed. Sleep induced by magnetism, and somnambulism, are also allied to states of insanity. Recovery may take the form of " awakening " but may also manifest itself as a prolonged battle.

In the general diagnosis of mental diseases, the following facts should be remembered: the ego, the personality, undergoes a change; it becomes estranged from itself, alienated. In order to be able to assess this, it is, of course, necessary to know something about the patient's previous personality. It is difficult to diagnose the disease process if its course is a slow one. It is also often difficult to differentiate it from borderline and transitional mental states and from ordinary eccentricity or immorality. Not everything that looks like mental illness is in fact mental illness. The diagnosis is made easier by a history of previous attacks, or by the absence of external causes. Insanity is primarily an abnormal reaction on the basis of internal causes.

The diagnosis should be based on the general impression of the patient, rather than on the presence of single symptoms. Beliefs in witchcraft or eternal damnation may be normal for one individual and pathological for another. Raving madness (mania) is characterised by excitement, melancholia by depression, and dementia by weakness of thought. Hallucinations, headaches, insomnia and convulsions may appear. All symptoms of cerebral disease are especially important in diagnosis. One must, of course, be prepared for simulation; since patients who are mentally ill in one way often resort to simulation of another illness. One will often be confronted with borderline states and one must differentiate between mental illnesses and typhus, intoxications and acute meningitis. Once he has made a diagnosis of mental disease, the clinician should always ask himself which part of the brain has been affected.

In order to determine the causes of insanity we must examine the past history of the individual, with respect to both his physical and his mental development. Mental illnesses are usually brought about by multiple causes. The seed of the illness is often laid down in that early period of life in which character formation begins. Several causes (such as shock, alcohol, worry) act on the brain and illness is then precipitated by a particular situation. Griesinger also still maintains the old distinction between idiopathic (which he calls protopathic) and symptomatic (deuteropathic) insanity.

Different nations appear to have different predispositions to mental disease. Griesinger believes that the increase of mental diseases is not merely an apparent one. The harmful effects of civilisation are, however, partly compensated for by the advances it promotes. Political influences are not a cause of mental disease, although they can be recognised in the content of the patient's deliria. He next discusses the effects of season, sex, age and social status. He points to the danger of imprisonment and particularly of solitary confinement.

Among the special predisposing causes he gives first place to heredity. Sometimes conditions are attributed to heredity which are, in fact, due to an upbringing which has been either too strict or too lenient (Ideler). Predisposing causes are also found in the psychic or somatic constitution, particularly in the " nervous constitution " which is characterised by irritability and weakness or by a hypersensitivity to psychological pain. As a result of many personal observations, he agrees with Fodéré and Lallemand that sexual difficulties in childhood may result in this type of constitution. He also mentions anaemia, shock and grief. How these causes act on the brain is unknown. He no longer believes in the great significance of cerebral hyperaemia which, until then, had generally been regarded as very important.

The most common causes are psychological in nature, and they are usually precipitating causes, or of fairly recent origin. Passions and affective states are much more often responsible than the notorious " intellectual strain." The first question Pinel always asked his patients was: have you recently had to suffer anger, grief or annoyance? If the conceptual complexes of the ego are seriously disturbed, conflict arises in consciousness and thus a split occurs in the ego. Psychological causes can act directly or indirectly via one of the organs of the body. Insomnia is a dangerous symptom.

Alcoholism must be regarded as a sort of mixed cause, since its effects may be physical and yet it may itself be caused by or give rise to grief. Dipsomania, that is periodic drunkenness, is a symptom and not a cause of mental illness. Sexual excesses also belong to the group of mixed causes. Masturbation may be harmless, but can also be a cause or a symptom of mental illness.

Among the physical causes Griesinger gives first place to other diseases of the nervous system, such as epilepsy, apoplexy, head injuries, nerve injuries, spinal neurosis or hysteria. Lack of sexual gratification, according to him, has been overrated as a cause of hysteria, since hysteria is quite common among married women. The physical causes comprise acute febrile illnesses and chronic constitutional diseases such as anaemia, tuberculosis, pellagra, and perhaps also diseases of the heart, gastro-intestinal and genital tracts. In the case of the latter, as also in menstrual disorders, it is often difficult to decide whether one is dealing with a cause or a symptom (of mental disease). In any case, the hospital doctor should carry out gynaecological examinations on his women patients. He himself had often cured hysteria in private practice by treating the uterus. Pregnancy and the puerperium can precipitate psychoses, but these are also dependent upon the predisposition and have a relatively favourable prognosis. Infanticide is often the manifestation of unconscious hatred.

It would, of course, be best to classify the mental disorders on an anatomical basis. Since this is, however, impossible, classification must be " physiological." (Here Griesinger uses the fashionable word of his group; in fact he goes on to develop psychological criteria). The beginning of the illness is marked by emotional disturbances without, or with only slight, organic changes. During the subsequent course of the illness, the emotional disturbances fade, and instead disturbances of thinking and of volition occur and numerous organic changes are found. Mental diseases are curable only in the first stage.

In this assumption of a single psychosis, with its two stages of development, Griesinger is following his teacher, Zeller; at the same time, however, he does provide us with detailed descriptions of hypochondriasis, melancholia, mania, monomania and feeblemindedness. Melancholia is a form of psychic pain. Almost all psychoses, in his view, begin with states of depression. Classical melancholia is characterised particularly by ideas of persecution and is related to hypochondriasis. In hypochondriasis, in which the patient's errors of judgment concern primarily his own state of health, we find a weak will and a feeling of estrangement. It appears to be due to abdominal or genital disturbances and to dyscrasia or psychological difficulties. In true melancholia, depression is followed by feelings of distaste and even of hatred for the outside world; by feelings of estrangement and by a withdrawal into the self. The patients may be silent for years. Guilt feelings play a major role and are followed by hallucinations with ideas of persecution and by catalepsy or states of agitation. Melancholia may change into mania (Falret), or into dementia and negativism. Suicide is a danger even in children. Incidental attacks of fever may be beneficial.

Mania may take the form of raving madness, recognisable by restlessness, impulsive behaviour and incoherence of ideas. In its alternative form of insanity, sensu strictiori, or " monomanie " as the French called it, one sees extravagant volitional states, with hallucinations, in the presence of an outward appearance of calm. The ego is here severely damaged and ideas of grandeur are common.

Griesinger subdivides the psychological states of feeble-mindedness into partial insanity, confusion (démence), apathetic dementia, idiocy and cretinism. Anatomical changes are frequently found in these cases. Cretinism, as Chatin has shown, is due to a lack of iodine in the soil. The chief complication of insanity is general paresis, as described by Bayle, Calmeil and Delaye. This is more common in men than in women. The second major complication is epilepsy.

The morbid anatomical findings in cases of mental illness are described in detail. Most abnormalities are found in the head. Pulmonary tuberculosis is very common. The prognosis depends upon the form and stage of the illness, and relapses often occur. Jaspers has listed Griesinger among the great descriptive writers; i.e., clinicians. His book, however, leads one to look for his greatness in another sphere, that of a man of ideas.

Treatment should be humane and not barbaric as in the past, but it could not always be mild. Physical and psychological methods must be combined and one must treat the patient and not the disease. Griesinger is a therapeutic optimist, and puts much emphasis on prophylaxis. He also believes in the importance of changing the patient's environment, particularly by separating him from his family, and by work therapy. The douche should only be used as a means of punishment. Instead he recommends baths, opium, digitalis, prussic acid and datura. He is opposed to the use of phlebotomy, blistering, purgatives and emetics. One should seek to recover and strengthen the patient's former ego. It is pointless to discuss delusions and one should divert the patient from this topic. Griesinger is a warm supporter of the system of " no restraint." Finally he discusses the problem, acute at the time, as to whether special institutions for the nursing of incurables (Pflegeanstalten) should be separated from hospitals (Heilanstalten).

Although in his youth he was exposed to the influences of the romantic movement, Griesinger, like the rest of his generation, was an anti-romantic and turned against both the psychicists and somaticists, whose contradictory theories he attempted to reconcile. He was an eclectic, but in a different way from Esquirol and his other French predecessors. His emphasis on morbid anatomy, and thus on the unity of psychiatry and neurology, is indeed very strong. He is the father of neuro-psychiatry, of the merging of the two disciplines, and his fame today rests on this alone. But he has more to offer: he presents us with a systematic synthesis of the anatomical, physiological, psychological and clinical points of view. All current trends in psychiatry can be traced to parts of his work. As a psychologist he developed Herbart's suggestions into such brilliant and apparently modern concepts as: the role of the unconscious; ego structure; frustration; and wish-fulfilment in symptoms and dreams. Herbart had, incidentally, also made a deep impression on Johannes Mueller and Feuchtersleben. Just as Marx claimed to have used Hegel's philosophy but at the same time to have " put it on its feet " (since, idealistically, it had walked on its head); i.e., to have interpreted it materialistically, so Griesinger might have said of himself that he had put romantic psychology on its feet.

The modern clinical approach is found in his view of mental disease as a process and not as a conglomeration of symptoms. This led him to adopt, from his teacher Zeller, the concept of a unitary psychosis (Einheitspsychose), with its stages of disturbed emotion and disturbed reason. He thus escaped meaningless exercises in classification. He still showed a full understanding of psychological causes. No psychiatrist before him had so consistently stressed the transitions from normal to pathological psychic processes as did Griesinger, who pointed to analogies, parallelisms and borderline states, sometimes using himself as an example. This is in part a result of his general medical theories about pathology as a form of physiology, but is in part also probably due to his personality.

The central elements of his synthesis consist of analogies with the latest neurophysiological observations on reflexes and inhibition. The reason for this is all too clear in view of his membership of a school of reform which called itself a school of " physiological medicine."

His synthesis no doubt had a liberating effect; following as it did on the dogmatic disputes between the somaticists and the psychicists. Naturally it was not free from gaps and contradictions. These were, however, apparently not noticed at all by his contemporaries. Judging by the effect of his book; which was almost exclusively to strengthen the concept of mental disease as cerebral disease, his great psychological contribution was either overlooked or misunderstood and, in any case, quickly and completely forgotten. It is hard to say why his synthesis was so much more effective than simultaneous attempts at synthesis made by Hagen, Sinogovitz and Feuchtersleben. It may in part have been due to Griesinger's literary qualities or to his personality. He was a strong reformer who also exerted much influence on the practical treatment of the insane. In part his acclaim may have been due to the general development of German medicine in his time, in part to the fame accorded him as a result of his University appointment. The change-over from institutional to university psychiatry begins with him and his pupils. Whatever the causes of his success, the fact remains that because of Griesinger, German psychiatry attained international repute and came more and more to dominate the international scene.

CHAPTER IX

BRAIN PSYCHIATRY AND THE CLINICAL SCHOOL

K. WESTPHAL (1833-1890), Griesinger's successor in Berlin, was a man with clinical, anatomical and physiological interests. In the clinical field he studied the obsessional neuroses, particularly agoraphobia, and perverse sexuality, which was also thoroughly investigated by Krafft-Ebing. In the field of anatomy and physiology his name is primarily associated, together with that of Erb, with the introduction of the patellar reflex as a neurological sign. From an organisational point of view, the period which was now to begin was that of " university psychiatry." Professorial chairs were established in Berlin in 1864, in Göttingen in 1866, in Zürich in 1869, in Vienna in 1877, in Heidelberg in 1871, and in Leipzig and Bonn in 1882. As far as its orientation was concerned, psychiatry was predominantly brain psychiatry. The most prominent exponents of this movement were Theodor Meynert (1833-1893), professor at Vienna, and Karl Wernicke (1848-1905), professor at Breslau. Meynert believed that every external stimulus set up a permanent state of excitation at a particular point in the cerebral cortex and that this was connected to corresponding nuclei in the cortex by means of association fibres. He held that psychological conditions correspond to such anatomical states. He also postulated that the cortex and sub-cortical centres were mutually antagonistic: diminution of cortical function results in a decrease of its inhibitory effects on sub-cortical centres and leads to hallucinations. Hyperaemia of the cortex results in states of agitation, whereas hyperaemia of subcortical centres accompanied by anaemia of the cortex produces a depression of mood. On this basis, Meynert created a comprehensive classification of mental diseases.

Wernicke was much concerned with aphasia; one of the three problems which, having been studied first in France, were now to be intensively investigated in Germany. The other two problem areas were monomania and general paresis, which will soon be dealt with more fully. Broca's discovery of the speech centre in 1861, whose existence had been postulated earlier by Gall and Bouillaud, once more raised high hopes of the possibility of localising psychological phenomena in the brain. Aphasia thus became a very popular field of study and, using it as a model, Wernicke drew up a whole schema of psychological disturbances. There is no doubt that Meynert contributed to the field of cerebral anatomy, and Wernicke must be credited with clinical achievements apart from his schema. Nevertheless, Nissl's designation of this movement as " brain mythology," and Kraepelin's as " speculative anatomy," were hardly unjust. Gudden, the old brain psychiatrist (murdered in 1886 by his patient, King Ludwig II of Bavaria; a common psychiatric fate in those days), surely had a franker approach to clinical questions, to which his standard reply was: " I don't know."

In 1857, Friedrich Esmarch and W. Jessen (*Allgemeine Zeitschrift für Psychiatrie*, 14: 20-36) for the first time suggested a connection between general paresis and syphilis and reported several cases. They thereby greatly advanced progress in the problem of general paresis in Germany. As a result of the neuro-anatomical orientation in psychiatry and of the advances made, particularly in Germany, in the technique of microscopy (Virchow), an enormous literature began to develop in anatomy and pathology. Up to now this has not yielded any final answers or practical results for psychiatry and, in this respect, has been largely unimportant and even worthless. The writings of Westphal, Gudden, Hitzig, Wernicke, Nissl, Alzheimer, Liepmann, Brodmann and O. and C. Vogt, however, have led to important advances in the sphere of pure science. To do justice to the brain-psychiatry of the nineteenth century, we must remember that a large proportion, sometimes perhaps up to 30%, of the mental hospital population consisted of paralytics; that is, of patients with demonstrable disease of the brain. Investigations also proceeded with much persistence, but few unequivocal results into other organic aspects of mental disease; such as blood counts, blood pressure, blood chemistry, body weight, temperature and urinary changes. A large series of diffuse classifications (Schuele, von Krafft-Ebing, Meynert, Skae, Maudsley, Tuke, Blandford) followed as a reaction to the unitary psychosis of Zeller and Griesinger.

Apart from these endeavours, which were in line with the vogue of their time, but were as a result of the special psychiatric situation largely sterile, the clinical school gradually began to emerge and was to reach its zenith of development in Kraepelin. The main aim of these workers was to delineate disease pictures, not by means of a classification of symptoms, but by means of observing illnesses throughout their total course. The attempt to get away from the symptoms as such was not new and can already be found in Pinel and his studies on the course of mania, but only now was it successful. In this connection, general paresis had served as a sort of model for a uniform type of evolution. But the successful elucidation of this and other organic psychoses, which resulted in their exclusion from the functional mental disorders, had left this field in complete chaos. Snell (1817-1892) was the first to attempt a formulation of new disease pictures. Stimulated by the problem of monomania, he tried to prove the existence of a third primary mental disease apart from melancholia and mania, which were at the time regarded as primary. This disorder he called " primary insanity " (1865). Westphal, Hagen and Sander, among others, did further work on " primary insanity " which finally gained public acceptance in the form of Kraepelin's " paranoia." Lasègue, in 1852, had already isolated a " délire de persécution " and Magnan, in 1883, had continued work on this subject. Karl Kahlbaum[1] became the most eminent pioneer of this movement[2] and from 1865 he was concerned with the delineation of what he called symptom complexes according to the model of general paresis. Ewald Hecker, his pupil, used one of these, the paraphrenias, for his description a few years later (1871) of hebephrenia. Cases of démence precoce had already been described by Moreau and Morel. Another such clinical picture was Kahlbaum's catatonia, which he described in 1869. Kraepelin's use of these two pictures as sub-groups of his concept of dementia praecox is well known.

Emil Kraepelin (1856-1928) graduated at Wuerzburg in 1878. He then became assistant to Gudden in Munich. In 1882 he moved to Leipzig where he soon gave up his neuro-anatomical studies with

---

[1] Karl Ludwig Kahlbaum, born at Diesen (Neumark) in 1828, graduated 1855 in Berlin. After 1856, physician at the mental hospital in Wehlau and Privatdozent at Koenigsberg. After his academic ambitions were shattered, he became director of a private clinic in Goerlitz in 1867. He died in 1899.

[2] It is one's task: " To build up disease pictures clinically so that as far as possible all phenomena manifested by the individual patient can be used to arrive at a diagnosis, and the total course of the illness is taken into account. The groups of disease patterns which thus emerge from study of the most commonly concurring symptoms, or from empirical delineations . . . were not only . . . easy to describe, they also led to a diagnostic approach which enabled one, far better than earlier classifications, to reconstruct very accurately the previous course of the illness from the present state and also to predict its further development with a high degree of probability, not only in general terms quoad vitam et valetudinem, but also in detail with respect to the various phases of the symptomatic picture." (Kahlbaum, K. *Die Katatonie*, 1874; in Jaspers, l. c., p. 474).

Flechsig and took up psychophysiological researches with Wundt. After holding mental hospital appointments in Munich, Leubus and Dresden, he became professor of psychiatry in Dorpat in 1886, in Heidelberg in 1890 and in Munich in 1904. In 1922 he retired from his chair so as to be able to devote himself entirely to the German Research Institute of Psychiatry which he had created. Kraepelin undertook several extensive journeys abroad; to Java, India, the United States of America and Mexico, in order to study mental diseases and administrative psychiatry in those parts of the world. He also became famous for his practical work; e.g., his fanatical campaign against alcoholism which was supported by so many prominent psychiatrists in those days, Forel and Bleuler among others. He exerted a decisive influence over the whole future development of psychiatry through his textbook, which appeared in one volume for the first time in 1883 as the " *Kompendium der Psychiatrie*," but which finally reached several volumes and attained its " classical " form only in 1899.

Even on the first page of his great work Kraepelin stated quite clearly that it is essential to know the clinical disease patterns, and that such knowledge could only be derived from observations at the bedside. He also stressed the importance of being able to make a valid prognosis which, incidentally, was often, according to him, a very gloomy one. He clearly recognised that pathological anatomy and experiments in localisation had failed to help in solving the problems of psychiatric aetiology. Despite this, he never gave up the hope that animal experiments, particularly with toxic substances, such as he had carried out under Wundt's direction, would have more to contribute in this field. The elucidation of basic physical changes would not, however, remove the need for psychological studies. Like others who in the course of medical history were not hopeful about treatment methods, he also stressed the importance of prevention and prophylaxis. Kraepelin saw clearly the social and legal problems in psychiatry. Among the aetiological causes known at that time, he distinguished between the external and internal causes. External causes, he thought, probably all acted by producing cortical damage. Here, unfortunately, all attempts at localisation had so far failed. As external causes he mentions intoxication, exhaustion, febrile delirium, metabolic diseases, alcohol, but also emotional upsets, although he accuses Griesinger of having made too much of these. A manic depressive state, he says, can for example occur with or without a previous emotional upset. He divides the internal causes or predispositions into general factors;

such as age, sex, occupation, etc.; and personal ones, particularly hereditary factors, which he considers to be very important, although here also the evidence is still uncertain. He dismisses stigmata. A faulty upbringing can, according to him, also result in a predisposition to mental disease.

After a general discussion of the manifestations of insanity (disturbances of the process of perception, of cognitive activity, etc.), of its natural history and of the methods of examination and treatment, Kraepelin describes the individual forms of disease as he has delimited them. In the present state of our knowledge, he says, the basis for this classification can be neither pathologico-anatomical nor aetiological, nor symptomatic, but must be derived from the total picture presented by the case material.

Kraepelin distinguishes between exogenous and endogenous psychoses. In the exogenous group he includes febrile deliria; psychosis due to exhaustion; intoxications, especially by alcohol; thyrogenous psychosis; general paresis; psychosis on the basis of a cerebral tumour or abscess, and dementia praecox. This disease picture, which he had created, in which he combined the hebephrenia and catatonia of Kahlbaum with a paranoid form described by himself, and which he defines essentially on the basis of its end state, he regards as being due to " self-intoxication." Among the endogenous psychoses he lists degenerative psychoses; manic depressive psychoses, in delineating which he draws upon the earlier descriptions of Baillarger, Falret and Kahlbaum; paranoia, which he created in connection with Snell's primary insanity; the neuroses (especially hysteria and epilepsy); psychopathic states (compulsive neuroses and homosexuality), idiocy and imbecility. One does less justice to Kraepelin than to any other author in such a short review of his basic theoretical ideas. His strength lies not in theory but rather in his descriptions of disease pictures. These cannot be reproduced in a shortened version and must be read in the original in order to lead to a full appreciation of his achievement.

Kraepelin had been a pupil of Wundt and he attempted to the last to base his work on the experimental method. He was, however, wise and unprejudiced enough to see that in the situation of his day the surest research tool in psychiatry was the clinical study of the natural history of diseases. On the basis of these studies he constructed the three fundamental forms of functional psychoses (dementia praecox, paranoia and manic depressive psychosis) as they are still recognised to this day, with which the reader will be familiar. Even today we are not yet in a position to say whether he had thereby created something of lasting value. But even at the present time we have to acknowledge that his work has lived longer than that of any of his predecessors. He has often been blamed for his emphasis on prognosis. Historically it would be just as unreasonable to make the same charge against Hippocrates and his pupils, who also laid great stress on prognosis. Surely it is already a great step forward if, in a situation in which he can neither arrive at an objective diagnosis nor offer any rational treatment, a physician can at least give a fairly accurate prognosis. Kraepelin was an eclectic with somaticist tendencies, which emerged especially in his studies on body weight, a subject investigated since the days of Esquirol, and in his emphasis on heredity. As a result, he was often inconsistent. One finds little discussion of psychology as such in his work and even less of psychotherapy. His limitations are nowhere so apparent as in his richly documented historical essay "*A Hundred Years of Psychiatry.*" In it he dismisses as out-dated not only the iniquities of his predecessors, but also their achievements. He had, however, great creative gifts and with these he assembled his many actual observations, like pieces of a mosaic, to form convincing disease pictures. This makes him, in our opinion, more than a " descriptive writer," as Jaspers called him in contradistinction to his " analytic " thinkers such as Wernicke. Kraepelin's work has proved to be surprisingly solid despite the harsh criticisms to which it was exposed, both at the beginning and towards the end of his active life.

This is largely due to later expansions and improvements made by others. Foremost among these was Eugen Bleuler (1857-1939),[3] who demonstrated the fact that dementia praecox did not by any means always end in dementia and who thereupon converted it into the schizophrenias. Here he introduced such useful criteria as Richtungs-prognose (general prognosis) and Streckenprognose (partial prognosis), which are similar to the general prognosis and Schubprognose (relapse prognosis) of Aschaffenburg. Bleuler also won great renown for transplanting Freud's theories of the unconscious into orthodox psychiatry. K. Bonhoeffer,[4] although highly critical of Kraepelin's

---

[3] Eugen Bleuler, born 1857 in Zollikon near Zürich. Studied in Zürich and Munich. 1884-85, assistant of Gudden, 1885 with Forel. 1886-98, Director of Rheinan Hospital; 1898-1927, Prof. of Psychiatry and Director of Burghölzli, Zürich. Died 1939.

[4] Karl Bonhoeffer, born in Neresheim, Wurttemberg, 1868: qualified in Tübingen, 1892; assistant of Wernicke in Breslau; 1903, professor at Koenigsberg; 1904 at Heidelberg and Breslau; 1917 at Berlin, where he retired in 1937. Two of his sons and two sons-in-law were executed after July 20th, 1944. Died 1948.

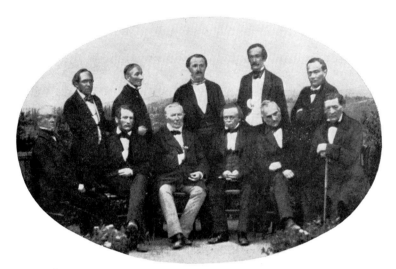

GROUP OF PROMINENT GERMAN ALIENISTS AROUT 1860

Standing: Dick.   Zeller.   Gudden.   Laehr.   Stimmel.
Seated: Damerow.   Kern.   Martini.   Roller.   Flemming.   Müller.

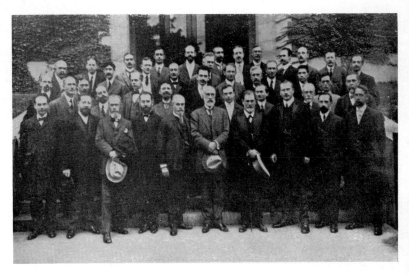

FREUD WITH DISCIPLES 1909

PSYCHOLOGY CONFERENCE GROUP, CLARK UNIVERSITY, SEPTEMBER, 1909

Beginning with first row, left to right: Franz Boas, E. B. Titchener, William James, William Stern, Leo Burgerstein, G. Stanley Hall, Sigmund Freud, Carl G. Jung, Adolf Meyer, H. S. Jennings. *Second row*: C. E. Seashore, Joseph Jastrow, J. McK. Cattell, E. F. Buchner, E. Katzenellenbogen, Ernest Jones, A. A. Brill, Wm. H. Burnham, A. F. Chamberlain. *Third row*: Albert Schinz, J. A. Magni, B. T. Baldwin, F. Lyman Wells, G. M. Forbes, E. A. Kirkpatrick, Sandor Ferenczi, E. C. Sanford, J. P. Porter, Sakyo Kano, Hikoso Kakise. *Fourth row*: G. E. Dawson, S. P. Hayes, E. B. Holt, C. S. Berry, G. M. Whipple, Frank Drew, J. W. A. Young, L. N. Wilson, K. J. Karlson, H. H. Goddard, H. I. Klopp, S. C. Fuller schema, developed his work further in the special field of the exogenous psychoses, particularly alcoholism. (Among the earlier important workers on alcoholism, besides Magnan we should mention Magnus Huss, 1849; Korsakoff, 1889; and Sutton, who described delirium tremens in 1813). An unexpected development; confirmation and enrichment of Kraepelin's work, was made by another of his critics, Ernst Kretschmer (born 1888). In his outstanding book, " *Constitution und Character* " (1924), he links two body types and two normal character types to the basic functional psychoses, schizophrenia and cyclophrenia (asthenic-schizothymia-schizophrenic: pyknic-cyclothymic-cyclophrenic). A contribution to diagnostic methods was made by the Swiss, H. Rorschach (1881-1922). His ink blot test (1921) stimulated the production of further " projective " tests.

The main aims of those who led the reaction against Kraepelin were to loosen his rigid system of classification and to enable wider factors not recognised by Kraepelin to be taken into consideration. The " Psychobiology " of Adolf Meyer (1866-1950), a Swiss working in Baltimore, should probably be interpreted in this way. The phenomenological school, both in its original form (" verstehende Psychiatrie "), as created by the psychiatrist-philosopher, Jaspers, and in its later form (L. Binswanger, E. Straus), which was much influenced by the philosopher Husserl, has no doubt contributed greatly to the understanding of the individual patient. Its reaction to the Kraepelinian system appears at times extreme (Jaspers: " Die Diagnose ist das Unwesentlichste "—" Diagnosis is of least importance "). Psychiatric phenomenology is of most significance for those with a philosophical bent.

Unfortunately, Hans Berger's (1873-1941) great discovery of the electro-encephalogram, so important in the field of epilepsy (1929), also failed to yield practical results in the field of mental illnesses as such. Traumatic (compensation) neuroses became a special problem for German psychiatry after Bismarck's (1884) introduction of national insurance. This problem has been intensively investigated there since the days of Westphal and of H. Oppenheim, the neurologist. It became particularly important during the first World War when the study of brain injuries also set new problems for psychiatry. Child psychiatry began to develop into a special subject as a result of the work of Moreau, Emminghaus (1882) and Ziehen (1894), although psychiatric illnesses in childhood had been recognised both before and since Pinel and Esquirol.

CHAPTER X

FROM NEUROLOGY TO PSYCHOANALYSIS

THE position of the psychiatrist about 1900 was not a particularly happy one. Although he was better able to classify the psychoses and predict their outcome than his predecessors a century before, he still suffered from the same ignorance of the causes of mental illness and he still had to be content with the same miserable methods of treatment. If he worked in an institution or a clinic, he saw only severe and hopeless psychoses, and although anatomy and physiology had been so helpful to his medical colleagues, they had failed to teach him anything about the nature of these illnesses, except in the case of general paresis. His patients were prisoners, and in a way he himself was a prisoner caught up in the difficulties of the field in which he had chosen to work. (From my own experience of the same situation, thirty years ago, I dare say that this is not an exaggeration). He was, to some extent, liberated from this situation by help from an unexpected source.

It is one of the great paradoxes in the history of psychiatry that neurology, which had at first served to strengthen somaticist trends in psychiatry, should now produce the pioneers of psychogenic research. Neurology had grown up. The enormous advances made in neuro-anatomy and neuro-physiology (Remak, Waller, Magendie, Marshall Hall, E. H. Weber, Dubois-Reymond) had been translated into clinical achievements by Duchenne, Charcot and his school, Brown-Séquard, Erb, Oppenheim, Struempell, Quincke, John Hughlings Jackson and Gowers. Most of these great neurologists were, incidentally, not " neuropsychiatrists " but " neurointernists." These methodical clinicians were also chiefly concerned with incurable diseases. But such diseases made up only a very small part of the material that confronted them day by day. Their consulting hours were crowded with people suffering from " nerves," and they were forced to do something for them.

In 1868, George Beard (1838-1882), an American, published his imaginative, impressive, lively and perceptive catalogue of the complaints which we now describe as neurotic, functional or psychosomatic.

He interpreted them on an organic basis as due to weakness of the nervous system, which he called " neurasthenia." In the seventies, the great Jean Martin Charcot (1825-1893) head of the Salpêtrière, who had achieved such enormous successes in the elucidation of tabes, multiple sclerosis and amyotrophic lateral sclerosis, etc., turned his attention to a functional neurosis, hysteria.[1] He studied hysteria as he had studied all other nervous diseases; by careful examination of reflexes, sensation, etc., with a view to finding evidence of organic damage in cases of hysterical anaesthesia, paralyses and contractures. He made observations on so-called hystero-epileptic seizures, on choreiform attacks and, above all, on " hysterogenous " ovarian pressure pain, which he regarded as a very specific manifestation of the disease. This gave scientific blessing to the operative removal of millions of ovaries from hysterical women by the adventurous surgeons of the period. According to Charcot, hysteria was a hereditary disease of the internal capsule, which produced " stigmata " and seizures, triggered off by the hysterogenous zones. Charcot's concept of hysteria was a tragi-comical misunderstanding. In the hands of his pupil, Babinski,[2] the innumerable specific neurological signs which Charcot had observed disintegrated and proved to have been largely based on suggestion.[3] Historically, however, this is of secondary importance, compared with the fact that because of Charcot's studies hysteria once more became " respectable."

From 1878 onwards, Charcot made further contributions in the field of the neuroses by his use of hypnosis in the study of hysteria (always on the same small number of chronic patients with severe hysteria at the Salpêtrière). Here, again, his methods were the same

---

[1] Jean Martin Charcot, born in Paris 1825, son of a coach builder. 1848, interne; 1853, Chef de Clinique at the Salpêtrière; 1872, Professor of Pathology and Anatomy; 1882, Professor of Neurology; 1893, died of a heart attack. World famous neurologist and teacher. Also very interested in the creative arts. His enormous library, now unused, is housed in a side room at the Salpêtrière.

[2] Joseph Babinski, born in Paris 1857, son of a political refugee from Poland. 1881, interne; 1886, Chef de Clinique under Charcot; 1890, Médecin des Hopitaux at the Pitié. Reflex studies, especially the Babinski reflex: neurophysiology of the cerebellum. Died 1932.

[3] Babinski's definition of hysteria was as follows: " L'hystérie est un état physique spécial qui se manifeste principalement par des troubles qu'on peut appeler primitifs et accessoirement par des troubles secondaires. Ce qui charactérise les troubles primitifs, c'est qu'il est possible de les reproduire par suggestion chez certains sujets, avec une exactitude rigoureuse, et de les faire disparaite sous l'influence exclusive de la persuasion. Ce qui charactérise les troubles secondaires c'est qu'ils sont étroitement subordonnés à des troubles primitifs." Babinski attempted unsuccessfully to replace the outmoded term hysteria with " pithiatisme " (curable by persuasion).

and his results erroneous. He considered hypnosis to be a pathological state which occurred only in hysterics and for which he invented a fantastic system of specific stages and phenomena. Here, also, the importance of his work lay not in his results, but in the fact that hypnosis, until then despised and neglected in academic circles— hypnotic phenomena were largely regarded as pure fraud—became not only a legitimate field of study and treatment, but for a time even an object of fashion because of its use by the greatest living neurologist and the most influential French physician. The studies in hysteria and hypnosis which now began resulted in the recognition of new facts, in the formulation of new theories and, above all, in undoubted therapeutic successes. These, whatever may have been their basis, once more destroyed the apathy and hopelessness which had begun to spread throughout the whole field of neuropsychiatry.

The following remarks summarise the early history of hypnosis: Franz Anton Mesmer (1734-1815), a Viennese physician, began in the seventeen seventies to obtain extraordinarily successful therapeutic results with a method which he called " animal magnetism," and which was also called " Mesmerism " after himself. Mesmer believed that the universe was filled with a magnetic fluid and that man's health depended upon its amount and distribution. Cures were achieved by a laying on of hands by the magnetist or through physical contact with objects; e.g. the famous " baquet," charged by him with magnetic power.   On account of constant animosity directed against him, Mesmer moved from Vienna to Paris in 1778. Here he at once attracted a large following because of his therapeutic successes, but he was also exposed to violent accusations of charlatanism. After being rebuffed by a Royal Commission in 1784, which consisted, among others, of Lavoisier, Bailly and Benjamin Franklin, he retired from public life to the Bodensee.

It was, of course, easy to refute Mesmer's naïve notions about magnetism. One fact, however, remained, although it may have been less important for the learned members of the various commissions which were concerned with Mesmerism in the subsequent decades than for the practical physician. This was that Mesmerism had extensive therapeutic successes to its credit. As a result, it did not depart together with its creator; on the contrary, it spread throughout France, Germany, Great Britain and the United States of America. It should not be forgotten that Mary Baker Eddy, the founder of Christian Science, had for years been a Mesmerist. In 1784 a pupil of Mesmer, the Marquis de Puységur, published observations on a sleep-like state which often occurred in the course of mesmeric treatment. This was the so-called artificial " somnambulism " which is identical with what today we call hypnosis. This is really the beginning of the history of hypnosis. As early as 1815 several French Mesmerists (Abbé Faria, Deleuze, Alexandre Bertrand, Noizet) realised that psychological (imaginative) and not magnetic forces were at play in this somnambulism and that it could also be produced without the laying on of hands. It appears, however, that this notion became more widely accepted only through the book of James Braid (1795-1860), the Manchester surgeon, which was published in 1843 under the title of: " *Neurypnology or the Rationale of Nervous Sleep.*" It is curious to recall that at the height of Mesmerism, numerous surgeons, particularly James Esdaile (1808-1859), who worked in India, performed often quite major operations painlessly under the influence of hypnosis. Braid coined the terms hypnosis and suggestion and explained the Mesmeric phenomena on a " physiological " (that is a psychological) basis. His phrenological notions, however, limited the value of his work.

The modern approach to psychotherapy sprung mainly from the work of the " Nancy School." Charcot's orientation had not been a therapeutic one. In 1850, Dr. A. A. Liébeault (1823-1904) had established himself as a general practitioner in Nancy, and as a result of the successful application of Mesmerism in several cases, he had come to the conclusion that the major factor in this was suggestion. Liébeault was a quiet man, a therapist rather than a theoretician, who only published his results in 1866, in a book entitled: " *Du sommeil et des États Analogues Considérés surtout au point de vue de l'action du Moral sur le Physique.*" This was completely ignored at the time. His methods were, however, studied in the eighties by the Professor of Medicine at Nancy, Hippolyte Marie Bernheim (1837-1919). He championed Liébeault's methods, attained good results from their practical application, and emerged victorious from a prolonged controversy between his school and that of Charcot. Bernheim, at first professor at Strasburg, had originally had a frankly somatic orientation, had been a pupil of Kuess and Virchow and a specialist for infectious diseases. In 1871 he moved to Nancy because he refused to continue to lecture at the University of Strasburg after it had become German. In Nancy he had no facilities (laboratories, etc.) for continuing his work in his usual manner and this was probably the reason why he then turned his attention to psychological methods of healing.

The publications of Bernheim and his associates attained tremendous popularity. From all over the world, young psychotherapists, such as Freud and Forel, pilgrimaged to the small and sleepy town of Nancy. It seemed that hypnosis and suggestion had at last provided a means not only of treating the neuroses, but also of investigating them. Neurotic patients were largely out-patients and psychotherapy did not necessitate hospital admission. Thus, just as in the seventeenth century, but for different reasons and with different results, psychiatry once more became largely a matter of " out-patient psychiatry."

In 1884, in the first edition of his " *Suggestion-therapy*," Bernheim described the methods of inducing hypnosis and said that it was not an hysterical neurosis as had been maintained by Charcot's school. He showed that their observations on hypnosis were based on artificially induced phenomena. According to Bernheim, almost everyone could be hypnotised. He regarded hypnosis as a state related to natural sleep. Just like deep sleep, the hypnotic state, he said, facilitated the carrying out of suggestions which, in the waking state, would be impeded by rational thinking, attention and judgment. He found no evidence for the transmission of anything physical during hypnosis, as had been assumed by the Charcot school. Braid had already proved that one is not here dealing with any " fluid." Bernheim considered that in hypnosis the patient was under psychological influence. In both his and Liébeault's experience, it was not sleep but suggestion which had proved to be the essential factor in treatment with hypnosis. The results achieved by means of hypnosis could almost all be obtained by means of suggestions made in the waking state, or by means of auto-suggestion.

Bernheim undertook numerous experiments in hypnosis; e.g., with post-hypnotic suggestion (already practised by Bertrand in 1823). This seemed to him to prove the existence of latent memories and to produce interesting and quite unrealistic explanations (later called " rationalisations " by Freud) of their behaviour on the part of the patients. He refused to assume an " unconscious " state, as experiences made during hypnosis can be recalled to memory. Bernheim produced in hypnosis even physical phenomena like blisters on the skin and hallucinations, which he called artificial dreams.

Bernheim's theory of hypnosis, which he himself described as being merely a formula, was as follows: Each human being is provided with numerous automatic (reflex, instinctual) behaviour patterns, which in fact predominate until the ninth month of life. Human beings are also, by nature, gullible and open to outside influences. Reflexes are normally controlled and inhibited by the brain, which provides a reasonable interpretation of sensory impressions. When this cerebral control is diminished, automatic and suggested responses are released. Despite this, the ego is not completely excluded in a state of hypnosis, but the reflexes come into action before it can take charge, since the state of consciousness is altered during sleep. This is also the basis of the " double life " (split personality).

Bernheim also examined in detail the implications arising out of this concept of suggestion for forsenic medicine (seduction, false testimony, murder) and for education. He showed that the effects of former methods of healing, such as the magnet, which had been used even by Laennec and Trousseau, of the healing touch of kings, and of places of pilgrimage such as Lourdes, were all due to suggestion. But as to what exactly suggestion was, and why it worked, Liébeault and Bernheim knew as little as we do today.

Bernheim treated mainly cases of hysteria, hysterical paralysis, neuropathies and neuroses (writer's cramp, enuresis). But he also had successes in cases of organic disease such as apoplexy, gastro-intestinal disorders, rheumatism, neuralgia and menstrual disturbances. Treatment, he said, must be adjusted to the patient. He analysed the causes of possible therapeutic failure.

These, because of the purely symptomatic nature of treatment with hypnosis, were bound to increase with time and to lead to disappointments and to neglect of the method from time to time. Up to now, however, we have always returned to it in certain circumstances; e.g., in both world wars.

We cannot here describe in any detail the golden age of hypnosis which ensued upon Charcot's and Bernheim's discoveries. Suffice it to say that hypnosis was not only used therapeutically, but examined also experimentally; e.g. in the work of Charles Richet (1875), Rudolf Heidenhain (1880), Preyer (1881), and that it was practised by such outstanding psychiatrists and neurologists as Freud, Bleuler, Moebius, Albert Moll, K. Brodmann and Oscar Vogt. (The latter subsequently attained fame mainly on account of their anatomical researches).

A wave of reaction against hypnosis and suggestion as psychotherapeutic methods began in the nineties, and the writings of the eminent German clinician Ottomar Rosenbach (1851-1902), proclaimed a method of treatment by persuasion and moral appeals. This " rational waking psychotherapy " (psychagogik) reached its height about 1900 in the work of the Swiss, Paul Dubois (1848-1918), who was joined by men such as Déjerine. These methods also were successful. Pierre Janet rightly and somewhat maliciously pointed out that the underlying principle of such methods, namely; to persuade the neurotic that his illness did not, in fact, exist, was suspiciously reminiscent of Christian Science. To what extent suggestion played a part in the successes of this treatment could never, of course, be exactly determined.[4]

The studies in hypnosis of the eighties brought a third eminent French research worker to the fore. He was Pierre Janet (1859-1947). Janet became Professor of Philosophy at a very early age and combined philosophy with a great interest in psychology. In 1889 he became established as a neurologist in Paris. In 1903 he was made professor at the Collège de France.

He had begun researches into hypnosis in the eighteen eighties[5] and had made the interesting discovery that traumatic memories, which the patient had forgotten, could produce neurotic symptoms and could hinder his adjustment to reality. Such memories could be discovered during hypnosis, and making them conscious led to cure. Janet published the first account of such cases in 1889. He is thus undoubtedly the father of what became known as the cathartic method of treatment. In his studies on hypnosis he came across the problem of splitting of consciousness, or split personality, and this he investigated intensively; as did A. Binet (1857-1911) and the American, Morton Prince (1854-1929).

Janet continued to use his cathartic treatment method, but only as one of numerous others. Although he too found that the traumatic memories of his patients often derived from sexual experiences and experiences in childhood, he warned against drawing universal conclusions from this. Sexual difficulties could in themselves be symptoms and not causes. One should fall back on the concept of the subconscious only if no better explanations for the pathological state of the patient emerged from his actual contemporary situation.

Janet regarded hypnosis as being parallel to natural somnambulism, that is as a dissociation of memory which enables other psychic tendencies to emerge. He believed that hypnosis could be induced

---

[4] For details see the excellent historical study, " *Psycho-therapie,*" by J. H. Schultz, Stuttgart, 1952.

[5] In describing Janet's point of view, I draw largely on his " *Les Médications Psychologiques,*" 3 volumes, Paris, 1919.

only in hysterics or in intoxicated people. He defined suggestion as a
reaction to certain perceptions: " This reaction consists of the more or
less complete activation of a tendency which has been provoked without having been completed by the participation of the total personality."
Suggestion artificially produces impulsions, that is the functioning of
tendencies which the patient was normally no longer able to produce
at will. Hypnosis and suggestion could release useful automatic actions
such as eating, sleeping, waking and recovery of memories. Janet
used hypnosis and suggestion with his hysterics, but he also used
education. He regarded hysteria as more than a phenomenon of
suggestion. For him it was an organic disease: " an organic split in
the compact mass of sensory perceptions."

Janet, like Freud, was of the opinion that the incidence of hysteria
was progressively declining and that it was no longer the commonest
neurosis.[6] Most neuroses, according to him, were not hysterical in
nature. They were based on exhaustion and fatigue and he grouped
them together under the term " psychasthenie." The symptoms of
psychasthenia; such as obsessions, phobias, fixed ideas, hallucinations,
depressions and compulsive behaviour, did not, according to him,
constitute the essential nature of the illness. They were all produced
by a lack of psychic energy, or tension, which lead to an inability to
carry out certain actions. States of emotional excitement arose from an
incapacity for adaptive behaviour, and states of profound exhaustion
and fatigue were the result of states of excitement, or of the inadequacy
and incompleteness of such adaptive behaviour. The patients become
" stuck in their actions "; they become compulsive. Janet adored econo-
mic metaphors. He talked of psychic capital, budget, etc., and said
that the most " extravagant " or costly form of adaptive behaviour
consisted of adaptation to one's job and to one's family. His intimate
studies of these problems (the mother-in-law, waiting, etc.) are highly
entertaining and realistic. He regarded social behaviour as being the
most complex.

Fear of taking action was one of the many symptoms which Janet
said could be interpreted as defence reactions, and it is for this reason
that rest and isolation have been found to be so beneficial for the
psychasthenic—and for his family. Because of his inability to love and

---

[6] The so-called decline of hysteria is perhaps explicable simply by the change
in diagnostic practices. Konrad Rieger, for instance, in his autobiographical
sketch (1929) said that some cases which he had diagnosed as hysterical in the
eighties and nineties of the nineteenth century, he would now call dementia praecox.

to command, the psychasthenic becomes dictatorial and longs to be loved. Impulsive behaviour (such as erotomania or alcohol addiction) provides the psychasthenic with a certain amount of stimulation. Janet reports remarkable cases in which depression was cured by kleptomania. Treatment should, therefore, he wrote, also provide stimulation, and suggestion contains an element of this. What is called physical treatment is often, in fact, psychological treatment. Many cases are resistant to hypnosis so that one's main task is to lead and to guide the patient. His confused situation must be clarified and he must be taught to live reasonably " within his small psychological means." Janet talks of educating, or rather re-educating, his patients. But, he says, this differs fundamentally from the education we provide for normal children, and from suggestion.

Janet was an accurate and diligent observer, a logical thinker and an immensely fruitful, versatile and interesting writer, who had a definite bent for systematisation. Nevertheless, he remained an eclectic. This deprived him of the drive and effectiveness of the dogmatist and system maker which we find in Freud.

Sigmund Freud (1856-1939) was undoubtedly the most renowned of all the psychotherapists and psycho-geneticists of the late nineteenth century. It is fair to say that in the first half of the twentieth century he was the most celebrated physician of his time, just as Paracelsus, Boerhaave or Virchow had been before him. He moulded the ideas which emanated from France into the form in which they became an international movement. In our brief review of his life and work, we are fortunate in being able to draw on the numerous, brilliantly written descriptions which Freud himself had published in this field.[7]

Freud was born in Maehren in 1856, but he grew up in Vienna. Anti-semitism flourished there at the time and he was forced into the position of an outsider at an early stage. In his early years he was mainly influenced by Ernst Bruecke (1819-1892); the physiologist and friend of Helmholtz, K. Ludwig and Du Bois-Reymond; in whose laboratory he worked from 1876 to 1882. Financial reasons forced him to turn to medical practice, but he continued with his neuro-anatomical investigations under Meynert who, he thought, was by no means well disposed towards him. At this time he was an extreme somaticist. He himself relates how one day, much to their conster-

[7] Particularly in " Die Medizin der Gegenwart in Selbstdarstellungen," published by L. R. Grote, vol. IV., pp. 1-51, Leipzig, 1925.

nation, he presented to his American students a patient with neurotic headache as a case of chronic localised meningitis

In 1885 Freud, then barely thirty, was made lecturer in neuropathology and obtained a travelling scholarship to Paris. There he studied with Charcot and became his translator into German. He then studied child psychiatry with Baginski in Berlin and in 1886 he established himself in Vienna. Freud is known to have conducted experiments with cocaine at this time, and it was only by chance that his friend, Karl Koller preceded him with the discovery of local anaesthesia. His reports on his experiences at Charcot's clinic (male hysteria and the production of hysterical pareses by suggestion) were met with disbelief by the Vienna Medical Association (" Wiener Gesellschaft der Aerzte ").

Disappointed in the then fashionable electrotherapy, Freud turned more and more to hypnosis. At this time he worked in close collaboration with Joseph Breuer (1842-1925), with whom he had become friendly when they both worked in Bruecke's laboratory, and who was an eminent neurophysiologist and one of the best known clinicians in Vienna. In order to increase his knowledge of hypnosis, Freud travelled to Nancy in 1889 and became the German translator of Bernheim. Since 1880 Breuer had observed that during hypnosis, hysterical patients can recall traumatic experiences, and that the reproduction of psychic events, repressed at the time, was therapeutic. Freud now began to use this same method of " catharsis," and he and Breuer published their results in an article in 1893, and in their book " *Studien über Hysterie* " in 1895: meanwhile Janet's relevant works had also appeared. In their book Freud and Breuer were still concerned to interpret their observations neurophysiologically. They called the transformation of the energy of repressed behaviour into symbolic symptoms " conversion," and the liberation of encapsulated affects " abreaction."

Shortly after their joint publication, however, the rupture occurred between them. Freud had gradually reached the conclusion that in all his neurotics; in cases of hysteria, of actual neurosis, anxiety neurosis, and neurasthenia, sexual difficulties were the cause of the illness. Breuer was not prepared to follow him so far. Freud also mentions a second reason for the rift. This was Breuer's adherence to neurophysiological explanations. Freud has perhaps never attached enough weight to the latter, and it is doubtful if he was ever fully aware of the decisive nature of the step which he now took.

Both Freud and Breuer had originally been neurophysiologists, and Freud also never gave up the idea that all psychological illnesses must, in the end, be attributable to neurological processes and that one day it would be possible to treat them causally with injections and pills. His later theories often still contained neurophysiological " models." In practice, however, because neurophysiological and anatomical research had yielded no positive results for the psychiatry of the neuroses and functional psychoses, he resolved to confine his work, first of all, to the purely psychological level. His great later achievements were possible only because of this courageous decision. Breuer, who was older and more deeply involved in neurophysiology, could not take this step with him.

Freud, at this time, also abandoned hypnosis as a psychotherapeutic technique and used other methods of recalling forgotten memories, at first those that he had learned from Bernheim. Only now did he become aware of the full role of repression in neurosis. Symptoms turned out to be substitute gratifications and the therapeutic task was no longer that of aiding abreaction, but of promoting the uncovering of repressions and their resolution by conscious decisions. Both Freud and Janet were concerned to enable the patient to adjust to reality. Freud called his new technique " Psychoanalysis."

In his study of his patients' unconscious, Freud became convinced that all neuroses are not only derived from sexual experiences as such, but from sexual experiences in childhood. He was only temporarily disturbed by the fact that his patients described scenes of seduction in childhood which later turned out to be fantasies. Freud now reconstructed childhood sexuality in its so-called auto-erotic, oral, and sadistic and genital phases. His explanation of neurosis as a regression to an earlier level of fixation of " libido " (his vague concept of sexual energy), as well as his concept of the " Oedipus complex," the kernel of all neuroses, stem from this period. His broadening of the concept of sexuality to include all pleasurable bodily functions necessitated the postulation of " sublimation." With this he had created a self-contained system; to doubt which was only the sign of repression on the part of the critic. As far as his technique was concerned, Freud now employed " free association " and began to study phenomena such as dreams and parapraxes in order to be able to interpret his neuroses. He recognised that the basic force in therapy was the phenomenon of transference, and he did not deny that this contained an element of suggestion.

For ten years Freud stood quite alone. In 1906 he was joined by Bleuler and C. G. Jung (born in 1875). The latter edited a psychoanalytic year book. In 1910, together with S. Ferenczi, they founded the International Psychoanalytic Association. A " Zentralblatt " was edited by Alfred Adler (1870-1937) and Wilhelm Stekel (1868-1939): *Imago*, a journal for the application of psychoanalysis to the humanities was edited by H. Sachs and O. Rank. In 1909 Freud held his celebrated lectures at Clark University in Worcester, Massachusetts, which brought him his first official international recognition. His way parted from Bleuler's as early as 1910. His two most gifted pupils, Alfred Adler and C. G. Jung, left him in 1911 and 1913 respectively, to develop their own systems. But despite this, the psychoanalytic movement continued to grow. Freud himself referred to his later writings after the first World War as speculative. These comprised, among others, his papers on the death instinct, " *The Ego and the Id*," and " *From the Pleasure Principle to the Reality Principle.*" Freud was influenced by Fechner early in his life but did not become acquainted with Schopenhauer and Nietzsche until later. In his later years he also investigated the psychoses, although these are not very accessible to psychoanalysis. Nor, of course, are they amenable to hypnotism. Freud also attempted to apply psychoanalysis to art and religion (Leonardo da Vinci, Hamlet, Totem and Taboo). In his late sixties he returned to general cultural studies, which had originally interested him much more than medicine (" *The Future of an Illusion*," " *Civilization and its Discontents* "). When in 1930 he received the Goethe prize, it seemed as if the furious hatred with which Germany had for years rewarded him for his achievements had, at last, subsided. Three years later, however, the all too familiar events took place which led to the death of Freud at the age of 83 as a refugee in London, in 1939.

It is clear that psychotherapeutic and psychogenetic ideas were in the air in the eighties of the last century. It was not by chance that Janet and Hack Tuke, in 1884, and Charcot, Déjerine and Freud in 1886, worked on so psychogenetic a subject as male hysteria. The reaction to the sterility of somaticism was unavoidable; the neurologists led it to victory because they had patients with whom one could work and make progress with a psychotherapeutic and psychological approach. The psychiatrists, who saw only psychoses, were, in this respect, confronted by a blank wall: Kraepelin had probably discovered more or less everything that could be learned at that time from psychotic patients in institutions and clinics. Later psychiatrists were able to apply to their psychotic patients the knowledge gained from the study of neurotics.

It is very easy to point to and criticise the speculative features—but had not somaticists like Meynert speculated in their time?—and other weaknesses of the psychogenetic trend, particularly of the Freudian system. It is also easy to predict that the pendulum will once more swing to the other side unless new basic discoveries are made to save us from the stereotypy of this movement. It is, for instance, quite clear that Freud had stretched the concept of sexuality far beyond its reasonable limits; that he had over-estimated the significance of child-hood experiences; that he was completely one-sided in his interpretation of symbols; and that the Oedipus complex, in the form in which he described it, was valid only for a particular social class in a particular place and at a particular period. Many of Freud's errors are probably attributable to his extreme determinism. He had taken this over from physiology, where it may be permissible—psychopathology, however, has hardly reached the stage where it is applicable. Freud's over-determinism to some extent explains his dogmatism. The latter made some of his pupils appear ridiculous, and he himself was saved from this only by his literary talent and his extraordinary intelligence. Freud repressed the fact that some of his ideas had been considered by psychiatrists in the first half of the 19th century. It is true that in contrast to his predecessors of the romantic movement, he was an empiricist and a materialist. It might have been better if he had acknow-ledged the work of his predecessors. As older ideas his inventions would probably have met with less opposition and he himself probably have viewed them more critically, instead of experiencing them as " revelations." The fact that in some countries psychoanalysis became a substitute religion; a church with all its paraphernalia such as pia exercitia (training analysis), etc., is a curious phenomenon which had, however, occurred before in other scientific movements, for example in Darwinism.

Moreover, it cannot be denied that the therapeutic achievements of the psychogenetic movement do not necessarily depend upon real etiological knowledge, or on causal treatment. It is to these achieve-ments that the movement owes its subsequent success. It would never have attained general recognition as a " pure science." The example of Griesinger supports this view. It is quite possible that the thera-peutic successes are essentially due to the same two basic mechanisms of confession and suggestion which are so little understood and which had been used with such success by the medicine man. Janet, appropriately enough, compared psychotherapy (excluding, of course, his own) with the mediaeval theriac, a strange concoction of the most varied drugs. If it worked, one never knew which of its many constituents had been responsible for the cure, and often one had to assume that the general effect was due only to suggestion.

It would, however, be unjust and historically incorrect to mention only the shortcomings of the psychogenetic movement and not its achievements. It is worth a great deal that many neurotics, and some psychotics, were actually relieved of their symptoms, whatever the causes of such improvement may have been. It was a great step forward, at a time when medicine was apt to be impersonal and mechanical, that doctors once more began to listen to what their patients had to say. Moreover, the psychogenetic movement liberated psychiatry from a state of hopelessness and sterility, and it cannot be denied that all psychiatrists of today, including the most sceptical and the most critical, have learned something from it. " Dynamic psychiatry " was no empty catchword. It represented an advance from the stage which Kraepelin had reached, of observing the external manifestations of total disease processes, to a stage at which such processes were to some degree understood. There is little doubt that at least a few of the mechanisms described will remain valid.

The increase in the vitality of psychiatry in the twentieth century was accompanied by advances in the field of preventive psychiatry. " Mental hygiene " had, of course, been practised by every psychiatrist from Pinel, Feuchtersleben and Griesinger to Janet and Freud. But it was the American, Clifford W. Beers (born 1876) who created the first organisation to further this campaign. He had written a very moving book about his own experiences as a mentally ill patient (" *A Mind that Found Itself* "), and in 1909, with the help of William James and Adolf Meyer, he founded the National Committee for Mental Hygiene in New York.

The so-called psychosomatic movement which developed in the thirties, whose aim was to investigate and treat the psychological causes of physical illnesses (peptic ulcer, asthma, etc.), came as a healthy reaction to the gross neglect of such psycho-physical relationships, which had occurred in the second half of the nineteenth century. It was a very valuable attempt, once more, to consider the patient " body " and " soul " as a whole. But the belief that something entirely new had thereby been created was historically naïve: almost every

great physician, from Hippocrates to Charcot, had been a " psychoso-
maticist," and the practice of expressing familiar or inexplicable
phenomena in a new and complicated terminology was a contribution
of doubtful attraction and value.

While the Freudian psychoanalysts had abandoned, at least temporarily, the search for somatic explanations, research in a very different
direction was being carried out by the famous Russian physiologist,
Ivan Petrovich Pavlov,[8] who quite deservedly won the Nobel prize
in 1904 for his work on the physiology of digestion. In the course
of his studies Pavlov had discovered conditioned reflexes, which are
controlled by the cerebral cortex and develop on the basis of un-
conditioned " natural " reflexes regulated by subcortical centres.
Pavlov differentiated positive, excitatory conditioned reflexes and
negative, inhibitory ones. The concept of nervous inhibition, familiar
since J. Budge (1843) and Volkmann, had been further developed by
the Russian, Setchenow, in 1863. Speed and concentration of excitation
in the cerebral cortex featured largely in Pavlov's explanations of his
experiments. About 1900 he began to substitute his " physiological "
objective psychology for the old-fashioned psychological psychology.
That is, he endeavoured to make conditioned reflexes the basis of all
mental phenomena. He even invented a " reflex of freedom." He
himself recognised the relationship between his aims and those of
certain North American psychologists, such as E. L. Thorndike (born
1874), and J. B. Watson, the father of " Behaviourism " (born 1878).
In 1918 Pavlov began using his methods to investigate psychopathology
and, particularly from 1928 onwards, his work lay predominantly in
the field of psychiatry.[9]

Pavlov was an outstanding experimentalist and his investigations
into sleep, animal hypnosis and experimental neuroses in dogs are
extremely interesting. However unlikely the assumption may be, the
idea that all mental phenomena can be resolved into reflexes has a
sinister attraction and points to an extraordinary breadth of vision.
We must here, however, limit ourselves to Pavlov's contributions to

---

[8] Ivan Petrovitch Pavlov, born at Rjasan in 1849, son of a priest of the Orthodox
Church. Studied natural sciences and medicine at the University of Petersburg
and qualified as Doctor of Medicine in 1879. Became laboratory assistant to
Botkin. 1884-1885, worked under R. Heidenhain and Karl Ludwig. 1890,
Professor of Physiology at the Military Academy of Medicine. 1904, Member
of the Academy. From 1921 obtained much government support (special Institute, etc.). Died 1936.

[9] Pavlov's psychiatric papers have been collected and translated into English by
W. Horsley Gantt, as " *Conditioned Reflexes and Psychiatry*," New York, 1941.

psychiatry, although for the sake of his reputation, we would rather
not have discussed them. But his psychiatry, together with the rest
of his work, has been raised to the level of a national religion in a
large part of the world and, therefore, we feel compelled to inform
our readers at least of its content.

In order to reconcile the contradictory results of his experimental
" neuroses " in dogs, Pavlov at first resorted to the hypothesis that
his dogs could be grouped according to the four " Hippocratic " temperaments ; choleric, sanguine, phlegmatic and melancholic, or, as
he defined them in his animals; excitable, lively, placid and inhibited.
His neuroses consisted of restlessness, whining, anorexia, and failure
to condition. They were produced by simultaneous inhibitory and
excitatory stimuli or by very strong stimuli in dogs temperamentally
predisposed to neurosis. These measures disturbed the normal
" dynamic stereotypy " of conditioned reflexes. In strong excitable
dogs, such stimuli led to a loss of almost all inhibitory reactions.
Pavlov at first called this illness neurasthenia, later hypersthenia. In
weak inhibited dogs, on the other hand, such stimuli lead to a loss of
excitability which Pavlov at first called hysteria and later neurasthenia.
This state could be improved by castration. While Pavlov assumed
that there were only two neural levels in the dog; the cortical and the
sub-cortical, he credited the human brain with a third level; the frontal
lobes, which contained the mechanism of speech. He distinguished
two basic types in man; the artistic and the intellectual. In the artistic
type, a coincidence of conflicting stimuli or an excess of stimuli leads
to hysteria; in the intellectual type, to psychasthenia; and in the intermediate type, to neurasthenia.

Hysteria manifests itself most clearly in dogs of a weak inhibitory
type. A weakening of cortical functions releases sub-cortical impulses.
If stimulation is continued, sleep finally sets in. Hysteria, according to
Pavlov, was chronic hypnosis.

Pavlov made extensive studies on hypnosis in his dogs. He regarded
sleep as a manifestation of inhibition. Hypnosis also was for him an
inhibitory phenomenon; an intermediate state between sleep and wake-
fulness. The spread of weak sensory impressions in the cortex produced
inhibition. A weak nervous system tired easily. Fatigue leads to
inhibition. Inhibition can also be produced by stimuli not translated
into action and by protracted stimuli. Strong stimulation results in
total inhibition in a weak type of animal. In hypnosis dissociation
occurs between motor and secretory functions, so that the flow of

saliva may be retained as a conditioned reflex response when swallowing movements can no longer be evoked. In hypnosis the cortex is paralysed while sub-cortical structures are still active.

Schizophrenia also is defined by Pavlov as a chronic hypnosis. For him it was the result of what he called the ultra-paradoxical reflex. He believed that he could observe schizophrenic symptoms, such as blunting, negativism, stereotypy, catatonia, in his hypnotised dogs, and that these also displayed playful behaviour, such as is found in cases of alcohol intoxication in which again the cortex is inhibited. Pavlov observed the same reaction in the ultra-paradoxically reacting animal. He regarded catalepsy as a paresis of the motor cortex due to what he called the cataleptic reflex. Catatonia was essentially defensive behaviour. On this basis he explained the success of rest cures and of bromides in his dogs. Certain experiments with his ultra-paradoxical phenomenon evoked " paranoia " in his dogs. According to Pavlov, one can initiate disease in certain parts of the brain without affecting the rest. He regarded senile dementia as a weakening of the inhibitory process in the cortex, due to age changes.

The reader will be able to form his own opinion on the somewhat doubtful value of these statements which, despite all their experimental foundations, were often very speculative and were also reminiscent of Meynert and Wernicke, who, however, had arrived at their formulations without troubling so many dogs. We know of no successful psychiatric application of Pavlov's " reflex psychiatry," Bromides, rest, or castration have not achieved therapeutic successes in man which Pavlov obtained by these means in his " neurotic " dogs. In order to use his results for psychiatry, a lot of reinterpretation seems required.

CHAPTER XI

THE NEWER SOMATO-EMPIRICAL TREATMENT METHODS

ALTHOUGH psychogenetic research had made some contributions to the understanding of the psychoses, it had unfortunately been largely unsuccessful in the treatment of this type of mental disorder. Fortunately a series of physical methods of treatment, which led to real improvements in psychoses, were empirically discovered in the twentieth century. We do not know, admittedly, why the methods are effective, nor have they appreciably contributed to our understanding of mental diseases; their effects have probably often been over-estimated and exaggerated. This should not, however, blind us to the fact that their use has resulted in the improvement and even recovery of numerous patients. In judging what follows, the reader should remember that almost all these methods are new and that many of their results have not yet been validated. Our assessment is, therefore, necessarily more in the nature of a contemporary opinion than of an historical appraisal, such as we hope we have presented in previous chapters.

The first successful physical method of treatment was discovered in the field of general paresis, the first psychosis for which an organic basis had been found. This was fever therapy. Ever since Hippocrates, it had from time to time been pointed out in the medical literature that intercurrent fever, and particularly malaria, occasionally results in unexpected recoveries in cases of mental disease, paresis or seizures. Similar observations had been recorded in cases of general paresis since 1816, when this disorder began more and more to be recognised. As a result, isolated attempts at treatment with artificially induced fever were undertaken in the eighteen-seventies. In a now classical article written in 1887, Julius Wagner von Jauregg (1857-1940), the young Austrian psychiatrist, discussed the possibility of treating general paresis with artificially induced febrile diseases, including malaria. The problem was an urgent one, because although general paralysis was now recognised as being due to syphilis, it failed completely to respond to the usual anti-syphilitic methods of treatment. A few years later, Wagner-Jauregg put his theory to the practical test. In 1890 he began to treat paralytics with Koch's tuberculin and later with typhus vaccine. He obtained some good results, but on the whole the method was found to be too unpredictable and uncertain to become generally accepted. In 1917 Wagner-Jauregg began to use malaria; in the course of the next few years he was so successful with this method that it gained general acceptance, and he was awarded the Nobel prize in 1927. Malaria treatment also yielded important results for malaria research. Although since the nineteen forties it has largely been superseded by penicillin, which is simpler to administer and produces better results, malaria treatment for progressive paresis remains a milestone in the history of medicine; not only because it led to a drastic decrease in the numbers of paralytics in institutions and prevented their rapid and certain downhill course, but because it naturally acted as an encouragement and incentive for further trials of physical methods of treatment.

One of the pioneers of modern physical treatment for the functional psychoses is Jakob Klaesi, whose introduction of continuous narcosis in 1922 must be mentioned. This never became a method of choice because shock therapy was introduced only a few years later.[1] Again, the fact that severe psychological or physical shocks can result in recovery from mental diseases had been recorded from time to time since the days of antiquity. Artificial shock had, therefore, been used repeatedly as a method of treatment.[2] Most people who employ modern shock therapy reject a comparison of their methods with those of the past. Some of the old methods, however, were so drastic that this comparison seems fully justified. The best known of the old techniques was sudden ducking or submersion of the mentally ill patient. This was practised from the time of the Greeks until the days of Boerhaave. It was Pinel and Esquirol who abolished it. The latter commented on this method as follows: " Lorsque je l'entends prescrire, j'aimerais autant qu'on donnât le conseil de précipiter les aliénés d'un troisième étage, parce qu'on a vu quelques fous guérir après avoir fait une chute sur la tête." (Esquirol, *Des Maladies Mentales*, 1838, Vol. I, p. 147). The method still survives as police torture. Just as drastic were prolonged cold showers and the various rotating machines which we have mentioned before. These also were for years

[1] Kalinowsky, Lothar. *Shock Treatments, Psychosurgery and other Somatic Treatments in Psychiatry*, New York, 1952. Sackler, Arthur M. Hay. *The Great Physiodynamic Therapies in Psychiatry*, New York, 1956.
[2] Buvat-Pochon, Christine. *Les Traitements de Choc d'Autrefois en Psychiatrie*, Paris, 1939.

reputed to produce good results until they were finally given up; whether for humanitarian or practical reasons it is impossible to say. The first modern shock therapy was insulin shock. Dr. Manfred Sakel (born 1900, worked first in Vienna, then in New York, d. 1958) discovered that marked psychological improvement occurred after hypoglycaemic coma and fits, produced by accidental overdosage of insulin, much used at the time for physiological reasons in cases of drug addiction. He now began to employ insulin coma and insulin-induced convulsions systematically in psychotics and was so successful with this that his method rapidly gained popularity. Sakel first used his method at the end of the nineteen twenties and published his first results in 1933.

Another shock or convulsive method; that of intravenous cardiazol, was developed independently by L. von Meduna (born 1896, worked first in Budapest, now in Chicago). Meduna began his investigations in 1933 and first published them in 1935. He started off from a false premise; that of the so-called antagonism between epilepsy and schizophrenia, and his aim was to cure schizophrenia by means of artificially induced convulsions. The first convulsant he tried was the traditional camphor. His results improved when he changed to cardiazol and this method rapidly became widely used after 1936.

After 1938 electro-shock began to replace cardiazol as a convulsant technique. Electricity had been used for mental diseases since the time of Perfect, but, of course, not in the violent form in which V. Cerletti and L. Bini introduced it in Rome in 1938. Shock methods were first used for schizophrenia and later for other psychoses, including manic-depressive psychosis; in which disease shock treatment seemed to achieve even better results than in the illness for which it was originally introduced. Despite this, many cases did not respond to it. Shock treatment was responsible for many spontaneous dislocations and fractures, the incidence of which was diminished by the introduction of curare by A. E. Bennett in 1940. Although their beneficial effects are recognised, opinion about these somewhat crude and brutal methods is still divided, particularly in view of our ignorance of the underlying mechanisms and the well known fact that spontaneous remissions and relapses can occur in the functional psychoses: it is still also open to debate whether their action is symptomatic or causal, and whether their effects are psychological or somatic.

" Psychosurgery " has not developed into a routine treatment, as have shock therapies. As early as 1890 the Swiss psychiatrist, Burckhardt, had ablated part of the cortex in mental patients with some success. Bechterew's pupil Puusepp (1875-1942) had severed fibres between the parietal and frontal lobes in 1910. But these methods had not become popular. In 1936, two Portuguese workers, Egas Moniz (1874-1955) and Lima introduced their prefrontal lobotomy, i.e. section of the white matter in the plane of the coronal suture, on the basis of what appears a somewhat primitive theory. The popularity of this operation is largely due to the energetic efforts of W. Freeman, an American, who adopted it at once in 1936 and modified it in several respects. Moniz was even awarded the Nobel prize in 1949. This operation undoubtedly results in improvement in some cases, but is, on the other hand, responsible for personality changes of such a degree that many people are still reluctant to use it.

All these methods now appear, to some extent, to be superseded by the latest advances in what is called " psycho-pharmacology."[3] Drugs have, of course, always been used in the treatment of mental disorders. Some organic psychoses respond to specific measures—endocrine disturbances[4] to hormones, pellagra to nicotinic acid, epilepsy to dilantin. Benzedrine and sodium amytal had a short period of popularity. Most drugs were, however, merely sedatives with their usual disadvantages of tolerance, etc., and they quietened the patient temporarily only at the expense of impairing consciousness.

In the alkaloids of Rauwolfia serpentina and chlorpromazine, we have found drugs which quieten the patient and yet, unless they are given in very high doses, do not impair his level of consciousness or his responsiveness. It had been known for about three hundred years that Rauwolfia serpentina was a drug used with success by primitive and other non-European peoples, but it had found no place in the European pharmaceutical armamentarium. Rauwolfia serpentina had already been used by the old Indian physicians and when, following the stimulus of India's political re-awakening, modern methods were used to re-investigate the old Indian drugs, Rauwolfia came to be studied in the early nineteen thirties by Sen, Bose, Gupta and others, who praised its efficacy in mental diseases and hypertension. In the early nineteen fifties it also came to be investigated in Europe and America, at first mainly as a hypotensive drug for use in cases of arterial hypertension. This action was, however, soon overshadowed

---

[3] Kline, N. S., Editor, *Psycho-pharmacology*, Washington, 1956.
[4] Bleuler, Manfred, *Endokrinologische Psychiatrie*, Stuttgart, 1954.

by its psychological effects (" ataractic," or " angolytic," i.e., diminish-ing states of anxiety).

At about the same time, the angolytic effects of chlorpromazine, a synthetic drug belonging to the anti-histaminic group, were being studied by French workers (1952, Laborit, Hamon, Delay, etc.). In 1954 it reached the United States via England and Canada. Since then these substances and numerous modifications of them have been used on a vast scale. How in fact they act we do not know. Numerous theories exist to explain their effects, such as that they act mainly on the thalamus, the hypothalamus and the diencephalon. The fact remains that they have a very calming effect without producing alteration of consciousness and that they often succeed in making even old and electro-shock resistant patients accessible to psychotherapy or spon-taneous recovery. Like all new drugs, they are probably over-estimated at present. They are, of course, not panaceas, and toxic side-effects occur. Their introduction has, however, meant that even the " disturbed " wards of mental hospitals have become quiet, and that it has been possible to cut down on the use of convulsant therapy. Hopes have thus once again been raised that they may point the way to more and even greater achievements.

INDEX